5K and 10K Training

5K and 10K Training

BRIAN CLARKE

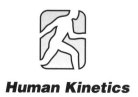

Human Kinetics

Library of Congress Cataloging-in-Publication Data

Clarke, Brian, 1955-
   5K and 10K training / Brian Clarke.
      p.   cm.
   Includes bibliographical references and index.
   ISBN 0-7360-5940-7 (soft cover)
   1. Running--Training.   I. Title: Five K and 10 K training.   II. Title.
   GV1061.5.C53   2006
   796.42--dc22

                                                    2005008530

ISBN: 0-7360-5940-7

The Web addresses cited in this text were current as of September 2005, unless otherwise noted.

Acquisitions Editor: Martin Barnard; **Managing Editor:** Wendy McLaughlin; **Assistant Editors:** Kim Thoren, Carla Zych; **Proofreader:** Julie Marx Goodreau; **Indexer:** Dan Connelly; **Graphic Designer:** Robert Reuther; **Graphic Artist:** Sandra Meier; **Photo Manager:** Dan Wendt; **Cover Designer:** Keith Blomberg; **Photographer (cover):** © Getty Images/Photo by Ian Waldie; **Photographer (interior):** Photos pp. 13, 37, 61, 77 © Human Kinetics; **Art Manager and Illustrator:** Kareema McLendon-Foster; **Printer:** United Graphics

Human Kinetics books are available at special discounts for bulk purchase. Special editions or book excerpts can also be created to specification. For details, contact the Special Sales Manager at Human Kinetics.

Printed in the United States of America   10   9   8   7   6   5   4   3   2   1

Human Kinetics
Web site: www.HumanKinetics.com

United States: Human Kinetics
P.O. Box 5076
Champaign, IL 61825-5076
800-747-4457
e-mail: humank@hkusa.com

Canada: Human Kinetics
475 Devonshire Road Unit 100
Windsor, ON N8Y 2L5
800-465-7301 (in Canada only)
e-mail: orders@hkcanada.com

Europe: Human Kinetics
107 Bradford Road
Stanningley
Leeds LS28 6AT, United Kingdom
+44 (0) 113 255 5665
e-mail: hk@hkeurope.com

Australia: Human Kinetics
57A Price Avenue
Lower Mitcham, South Australia 5062
08 8277 1555
e-mail: liaw@hkaustralia.com

New Zealand: Human Kinetics
Division of Sports Distributors NZ Ltd.
P.O. Box 300 226 Albany
North Shore City
Auckland
0064 9 448 1207
e-mail: info@humankinetics.co.nz

In memory of Arthur Lydiard (1917-2005).

Contents

Preface

Every runner has a story, and every training program forms another chapter in that story. Some runners train to set a personal record in a goal-race; others simply want to get in better shape than last year. Whatever your personal goal, a successful story should include effective, individualized training.

Unless your training fits your individual needs and goals, it's unlikely your programmatic story will result in the running of a successful goal-race. The programs and discussions in this book will give you the tools to know when you are running too hard, too easy, or just hard enough for injury-free training and improved racing performances.

This book is not a quick-fix compendium of tips for 5K and 10K training. Rather, it's an integrated system for dealing effectively with the complexities of the training process. By learning and using the tenets of the hard–easy system, you can solve the perennial problems inherent to endurance training, including knowing *when* and *how hard* to train.

I've been in the game of competitive running since 1961. I've directed training and educational programs for recreational runners and triathletes since 1979. I learned the hard–easy system from Bill Bowerman–one of the premier track coaches of the 20th century. Over the years I've worked with athletes of all levels, and I know that a variety of runners can benefit from the training programs outlined here. Beginners can use this book as a training primer. Intermediate and advanced athletes will value its solutions to the recurrent training problems.

Chapters 1 through 4 contain the background information you'll need to understand how a training program works by defining the five racing abilities–stamina, power, tempo, speed, and endurance–and providing scales for gauging how hard you are working so you can run optimal workout efforts. They also provide questionnaires to determine your current capacity for exertion so you can adjust new workouts to that capacity without becoming sick or injured at the outset.

Chapters 5 through 9 describe the process of creating a training program, including descriptions of seven new workouts with instructions on establishing and building ability with them. Also included are sample training programs for 5K and 10K races, as well as a unique effort–energy training log for recording your workouts and tracking your progress.

The guidelines set forth in this book will teach you to coordinate your workout effort with your running energy for ability-building purposes. They will also assist you in targeting and monitoring your exertion so you can accomplish your racing goals. By following the programs in *5K and 10K Training* you will be able to train smarter and perform better so you can live a happy running story.

Acknowledgments

Many readers have asked me whether I research my books. I don't research them as much as I think about how to solve various problems. My thinking is inseparable from my writing, and I never research what others have said on a topic while I'm writing.

My first book helped me to define the major constructs of effort and energy. In my second book, *Running by Feeling* (1999), I used previously developed concepts to survey the recurring problems of endurance training. The current book focuses on setting up new ability-building workouts, and how those workouts fit into a training program. In this regard, I'm indebted to my editors at Human Kinetics for encouraging me to think programmatically.

While writing this book, I had several conversations with Nobby Hashizume, a protégé of Arthur Lydiard. I knew Lydiard personally from the early 1960s when he stopped in Honolulu for track meets with his New Zealand athletes. During those visits, he gave clinics on the training process that influenced me to take my first 20-mile training runs. Lydiard also had a major effect on my track coach at the University of Oregon, Bill Bowerman. Hashizume reminded me of Lydiard's enormous contribution to my understanding of endurance training.

My thinking and writing are footnotes to the ideas developed by Bowerman and Lydiard. Bowerman taught me about the hard–easy system, structuring exertion to build ability, and the peaking process. I've taken his ideas and added perspective, but there is nothing fundamentally new here that wasn't already said by Bowerman and Lydiard.

CHAPTER 1

Understanding Effort and Energy

This book describes the role that effort and energy play in training for 5K and 10K races. Effort and energy are the essential aspects of every run. You cannot do a race or a workout without exerting an effort or encountering running energy.

Effort and energy are also the building blocks of adaptation. This chapter introduces you to the idea of effort so you can gauge your training effort for ability-building purposes. It will also help you understand how changes in your running energy determine how much effort you should exert during the training process.

Reading Body Language

5K and 10K Training is based on the premise that you can read your body to tell when you are running too hard, too easy, or just right. Suppose you needed to run a workout at 65 percent of your maximum heart rate. How would you know when you had it right?

If you knew your maximum heart rate and you had a heart rate monitor, it would be easy to get it right. But if you had to rely only on the experience of your beating heart, it would be difficult to tell. This is because your heartbeat is not usually a conspicuous part of your experience.

Fortunately, we don't have to rely exclusively on heartbeat to measure exertion, because exercise exertion consists of five components, including heart rate, breathing, power, tempo, and intensity (see table 1.1).

TABLE 1.1   Five Components of Perceived Exertion

Heart rate	Breathing	Power	Tempo	Intensity
95-100%	Hyper	Strained	Very fast	Very uncomfortable
90-94%	Labored	Forced	Fast	Uncomfortable
80-89%	Heavy	Pressed	Rapid	Tolerable
70-79%	Huffing	Relaxed	Quick	Comfortable
60-69%	Conversational	Held back	Slow	Very comfortable
50-59%	Normal	Gentle	Very slow	Soothing

Separately, these components of perceived exertion are useful for recognizing how exertion changes from moment to moment during a run. Each component is a distinct and recognizable experience: Heart rate is the per-minute rate at which your heart is beating; breathing is the rate at which you inhale and exhale; power is the sense of muscle strength you are applying to a run; tempo is the rate at which your arms and legs are moving; and intensity is your relative sense of comfort or discomfort.

Each component of exertion is scaled into six levels. Most of the time, the experience of one component is related to the experience of the others at the same level. Thus we can talk about six general levels that I call mild, light, steady state, threshold, ragged edge, and maximum.

Defining the Six Levels of Exertion

Everyone is capable of a wide range of exertion, from the slowest jog to the fastest run. In this sense, exertion is the physical effort necessary to sustain a pace from moment to moment during a run. Exertion is also the essential adaptive stimulus. You can't build your racing ability without exerting an effort.

To get the most out of your training, you must learn to distinguish between the various levels of exertion, using each level purposefully to train and race effectively. The following material will describe the six exertion levels in more detail.

> **Mild**. Mild exertion can be defined as your slowest jogging pace. Your heart rate at that pace will be 10 to 15 beats per minute faster than your heart rate at a brisk walk, even though both paces are the same in minutes per mile. This increase in heart rate reflects the additional effort required to get airborne between jogging steps—effort you don't exert while walking.

Some athletes are unwilling to run at their slowest pace. They overlook the value of a very slow glide, which is useful in a variety of circumstances. When you're injured, for example, gentle jogging may allow you to continue exercising without causing further injury. Very slow jogging also conserves energy while warming up before a race or workout or when you are recovering from a particularly tiring run.

Fast runners are often uncomfortable running at mild exertion because they feel awkward and inefficient at their slowest pace. They lumber along, overstriding to the point of walking instead of jogging. If you want to be efficient at your slowest jog, take short, quick steps, and repeat the following mantra, "Short and quick; short and quick," matching the tempo of your feet to the tempo of the mantra.

Taking little steps feels strange at first, but learning to be efficient at your slowest pace can broaden your training range by giving you a valuable extra level of exertion.

> **Light.** Although light exertion feels slow, it represents a relatively high level of metabolic activity: roughly 60 to 69 percent of your maximum heart rate, which is approximately double your resting heart rate.

Most trained endurance athletes who are running at 60 to 69 percent of maximum experience exertion as conversational breathing at a very comfortable, slow tempo that feels "held back" in the sense that they would have to consciously prevent themselves from moving at a faster pace.

Like the mild level, light exertion enables you to run for a long time. As you'll see, long duration runs are the base upon which faster running is built.

> **Steady State.** Steady state is the level between 70 and 79 percent of maximum heart rate. At that level your tempo feels quick and relaxed, with deep, slow, inaudible breathing and a discernable "huff" between phrases of conversation.

Huffing is not necessarily an indication of being out of shape. Even the best athletes huff when exerting themselves at steady state. With proper training, all athletes eventually get in shape and move at a relatively faster pace when they are running at steady state.

> **Threshold.** The threshold level is characterized by audible, heavy breathing at a rapid, pressed tempo. Most runners encounter audible breathing between 80 and 89 percent of maximum heart rate. At that level they are no longer merely huffing between sentences of more-or-less normal conversation, but breathing loud enough for someone running next to them to hear each exhalation. Threshold exertion precludes "normal" conversation because it requires focused concentration to maintain the pace.

> **Ragged Edge.** The ragged-edge level is a fast, forced tempo, with labored breathing and intense discomfort at 90 to 94 percent of maximum heart rate. Only the most courageous athletes push themselves hard enough to explore exertion between 90 and 100 percent of maximum. Even at the lower half of this range, ragged-edge exertion is downright uncomfortable. While some athletes can sustain ragged-edge exertion without apparent distress, it's almost impossible to conceal some enabling emotion.

> **Maximum.** Maximum exertion running is at the opposite end of the scale from very slow jogging. Most runners can reach maximum exertion at the finish of a highly competitive 5K race. At maximum exertion—95 to 100 percent of maximum heart rate—breathing is hyper fast and you strain to maintain the pace against the onslaught of extreme discomfort and inexorable fatigue.

TARGETING EXERTION ON THE EDGE

Sometimes when I'm running intervals at the border between steady state and threshold, I find myself pressing instead of relaxing. Even though my heart rate is technically still within my steady-state level, I grip my stopwatch tightly, grimace slightly, and, of course, I press the pace instead of being relaxed in spite of it.

At times like those, I have to remind myself to stay relaxed. After all, the target zone is still ostensibly steady state, even though I'm aiming for the upper edge of it. This example points out the problem of exertion levels blending with one another at their borders. This is an unavoidable aspect of measuring perceived exertion. Nonetheless, a cogent scheme for measuring exertion should delineate reasonable, yet clearly differentiated, levels—even though the characteristics of one level tend to blend at the border with the characteristics of the adjacent level.

As long as an exertion level is delimited by characteristics that make it distinct from adjoining levels, there is still reason to use the measuring scheme because it squares with our experience. After all, we are only talking about a conceptual measuring tool, and the true value of such a tool is its utility.

Calculating Maximum Heart Rate

According to this scheme, exertion is cut into increments of 5 or 10 percent. I could have made the exertion levels wider or narrower, but these particular levels are wide enough that the perception of exertion at each level changes in regular, distinct, and noticeable fashion as exertion increases in intensity.

I recommend memorizing each exertion level so you can recognize how hard you are working at any moment of a run. This is an introspective, subjective process. But once you know your maximum heart rate, you can use a heart rate monitor to measure your exertion more objectively. Before you can use this method, however, you need an accurate measure of your maximum heart rate.

The most reliable way to accurately determine your maximum heart rate is to take a reading while running at maximum exertion. You could record your heart rate near the end of a highly competitive 5K race. Or you could test yourself using the following protocol.

You'll need a heart rate monitor for this test. If your monitor doesn't store data for later retrieval, you can station a couple of friends with clipboards and stopwatches at 200-meter intervals on a 400-meter track. Hold the monitor in your hand so you can easily see the readout and, as you pass your friends, yell out your heart rate so that they can record it along with your split times.

You should have abundant energy for this test. It's difficult to run all-out when you are tired from recent training. So give yourself enough rest that you can raise your heart rate to its true maximum. Please refer to the box on page 6 for the HR protocol test.

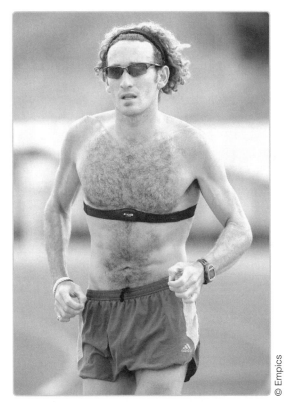

The band on the runner's chest transmits data to the heart rate monitor on his wrist.

Measuring Workout Effort

As you'll soon see, adaptation depends on how you coordinate measured workout efforts with your variable sense of energy. The first concept you'll need to grasp in order to build your racing ability is workout effort. Two simple words, but do you have a clear understanding of their meaning? Since many runners confuse workout effort and exercise exertion, our first task is to make a clear distinction between these important concepts.

Exertion, as you have already seen, tells you how hard you are working from moment-to-moment within a race or workout. Workout effort, by contrast, is a measure of the difficulty of a whole run, including all its exertion moments. The longer you run at any given heart rate, the harder the overall workout becomes. With workout effort, it's the overall effect of exertion that counts. Thus, a long-duration workout can be a hard workout even though the pace felt "easy" (light) the whole way.

TESTING FOR MAXIMUM HEART RATE

Warm-up
Begin at your slowest jogging pace. After 15 minutes of very slow jogging, do several 50-meter pickups, building to a quick, relaxed pace.

Test
When you are completely warmed up, begin a six-lap, nonstop test, recording your heart rate and split times every 200 meters.

1. Run laps one and two at a quick, relaxed pace (steady state). Your breathing should be inaudible to someone running beside you.
2. Run laps three and four at a rapid tempo, pressing the pace (threshold). You should begin to hear your breathing after a lap at this level, but it should not be labored—merely noticeable to someone running beside you.
3. Run lap five and the first half of lap six at your fastest sustainable pace—fast enough to cause ragged, labored breathing (ragged edge), but not so fast that you cannot accelerate during the last half lap.
4. Run the last 100 to 200 meters as fast as you can (maximum). Be sure to check your heart rate monitor at the finish, as that will be your maximum.

Cool-down
Jog a lap or two at your slowest jogging pace and notice how quickly your heart rate drops from its highest level. Jogging very slowly after a race or workout helps to dissipate lactic acid and speed recovery.

Here's a thought problem for you: Suppose you were scheduled to run a hard workout. How would you know when you've run a hard workout, rather than a moderate or a very hard one? This is an important question because effective training requires that you gauge your effort exactly for ability-building purposes.

If you were scheduled to run a hard workout, you should be able to end the workout without over- or undertraining. And having just completed the workout, you should be able to say exactly how hard it was, whether relatively hard or easy. Gauging your workout effort is an intuitive skill that's necessary as a check on momentary whim. Running by feeling is not the same as running by caprice.

A defining characteristic of any effort is the fatigue that sets in as you exert it. All workouts—even the easiest—cause some fatigue, but noticeable fatigue is one of the delimiting marks of a hard workout (see table 1.2). Table 1.2 describes the fatigue generated by five different levels of workout effort. The harder a workout, the more fatigue it generates. This fatigue is distinct from your fatigue going into the workout. Thus, a very easy workout generates imperceptible fatigue, but you may have been already fatigued from other recent workouts. Noticeable fatigue usually comes on gradually as your efficiency disintegrates, your energy flags, your joints become achy, and your legs become heavier and less responsive.

TABLE 1.2　The Fatigue Generated by Five Workout Efforts

Effort	Level of fatigue
Very Easy	Imperceptible and insignificant
Easy	Perceptible, but negligible
Moderate	Appreciable, but minor
Hard	Noticeable and significant
Very Hard	Obvious and major
All-Out	Strikingly evident, overwhelming

So the question is, how would you know when you've run a hard workout? First, you can simply intuit the difficulty of the effort based on your experience of its intensity and duration. By this method, when you finish a hard workout you'd say, "Whew, that was a *hard* workout." By contrast, a moderate workout would feel only moderately difficult, and a *very* hard workout would be a killer.

Second, even if you weren't sure how difficult a workout was when you finished, you'd know by seeing how long it takes to recover from it. If your recovery takes 24 to 36 hours, it was a moderate workout. If it takes between 48 and 60 hours, it was a hard workout; if it takes longer than 60 hours it was at least a very hard workout.

At this point you should have a conceptual grasp of workout effort and, in that context, the following workout effort scale should make some sense to you.

Workout Effort Scale

Very Easy: A very easy workout is very short and very slow. You recover from a very easy workout in less than 12 hours.

Easy: An easy workout is short and slow. You recover in about 12 hours.

Moderate: A moderate workout can be short and quick or somewhat longer and slower. You need 24 to 36 hours to recover from a moderate workout.

Hard: A difficult, noticeably fatiguing workout that can be relatively long and slow, or short and fast. It takes 48 to 60 hours to recover from a hard workout.

Very Hard: A very difficult race or workout. It can be very long and slow, or shorter and faster, but the key factor is major fatigue. Most conditioned athletes need at least 72 to 84 hours to recover from a very hard workout.

All-Out: You've run all-out when you couldn't have run faster for the distance, or longer without slowing down. Most all-out efforts take more than 84 hours for recovery, but some all-out races can take one day of recovery for every racing mile.

I have used the ideas of fatigue and recovery to delimit different levels of workout effort. Technically speaking, however, fatigue and recovery belong to another conceptual construct–namely energy. To better understand workout effort you should also understand running energy, which is the subject of the next section.

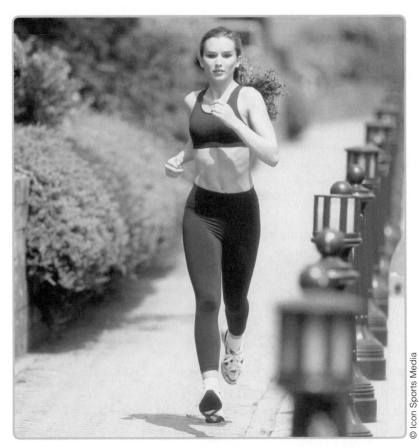

You should be ready for your hard workouts; your level of energy should be sufficient for the difficulty of the effort.

Measuring Running Energy

Whenever you exert a running effort you push against your internal, metabolic resistance to effort, that is, energy. If you happen to have a lot of energy, your effort encounters little resistance and you feel like you're flying. But when you are out of energy even an easy run can be tough to do.

Fortunately, you don't need a special monitor to measure your running energy. All you have to do is take a run and feel it on the following scale: no energy, little energy, some energy, ample energy, and abundant energy. This scale measures your running energy as you feel it *in the moment*.

The interesting thing about running energy is the way it can change from moment to moment during a run. Most runners have noticed, for example, how they can start off with only some energy, but after awhile they develop ample energy—even enough for a hard workout. This changeability of energy is a quality of its cyclic nature.

Left to follow the metabolic forces that govern it, your energy always moves through several phases from the start of one workout to the start of the next. Each phase changes the amount of energy you experience, first by contracting your energy, then by expanding it. These fluctuations in the amount of energy you experience form an energy cycle that's common to most workouts (see figure 1.1).

There are two ways you can understand your energy: as running energy and as workout energy. Because running energy typically changes during a run, workout energy is actually a measure of the *pattern* of running energy that develops during a whole workout.

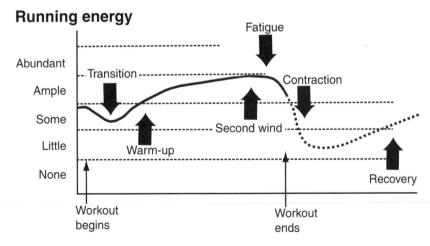

Figure 1.1 The arrows (representing metabolic forces) cause running energy to fluctuate during a run. Given enough time between workouts, the recovery force will return running energy to the original level. This is the basic energy cycle for all runs.

The specific energy pattern illustrated in figure 1.1 is ready-to-run-hard. It is characterized by some energy at the start of a workout, which develops into ample energy after a 10- or 15-minute warm-up. Ample energy is usually sufficient to accommodate a hard workout, meaning a difficult, noticeably fatiguing workout that requires 48 to 60 hours of recovery time.

Experienced runners can say which pattern of energy will develop during a run based on how their running energy develops during the first few minutes. The ability to make this distinction is one of the most important skills in running, for being successful in the competitive game depends on coordinating your training effort with your fluctuating sense of energy.

Understanding the Five Workout Energy Patterns

Ready-to-run-hard is one of five workout energy patterns called sluggish, tired, lazy, ready, and eager. Each pattern is distinct from the others, as described in the following definitions and seen in figure 1.2.

Running energy

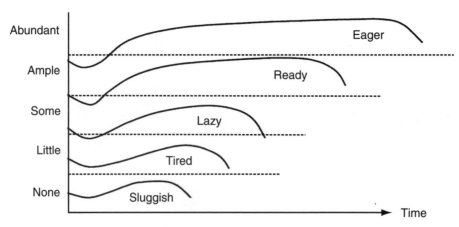

Figure 1.2 Running energy fluctuates within a workout as shown in this figure illustrating five different workout energy patterns. Each pattern represents the typical flow of energy during a single workout, depending on how much energy you had to start. The patterns range from sluggish (no energy and it never gets better) to eager (abundant energy develops early and lasts a relatively long time).

Workout Energy Scale

Eager-to-Race: Abundant energy and an aggressive attitude are sustainable at a racing pace.

Ready-to-Run-Hard: Ample energy develops after a short warm-up, and it lasts long enough for a hard workout.

Too-*Lazy*-to-Run-Hard: Little energy at the start. Some energy develops slowly–perhaps even to ample energy–but it runs out early.

Too-*Tired*-to-Run-Moderate: A little energy can develop, but you cannot run harder than a short, slow workout without being burdened by the effort.

Too-*Sluggish*-to-Run-Easy: You have no energy from start to finish of a run. You feel terrible for the whole workout.

You can never predict exactly what energy pattern will develop during a run. It depends on the difficulty of recent workouts, the length of your last recovery period, the amount of sleep you've had recently, the quality of the food you've eaten, and your mental preparation for the effort.

Similarly, you can have slightly more or less starting energy than any of the five energy patterns described in the workout energy scale. You can also expect the five patterns to develop in slightly different ways, depending on your starting energy. With practice, as you experience different levels of energy and you become skilled at measuring them, you should be able to distinguish gradations between workout energy patterns.

When it comes to energy, the goal is to have enough of it to do a scheduled workout. Since you cannot produce energy on demand, you've got to know how to control it indirectly, with effort. In other words, to control your energy you have to control your effort. And, conversely, the only way you can optimize training effort is to give absolute priority to your energy.

It follows that energy is not an arbitrary factor that sometimes hinders performance and sometimes enables it. Rather, energy should be the central focus of the training process. It doesn't matter how many miles you plan to run during a certain workout. The only thing that matters is whether you have the energy to run those miles.

Optimizing Workout Effort

Every thoughtful runner has dealt with the question of how to optimize workout effort. With six levels to choose from, the answer isn't necessarily apparent. For instance, which of the following levels of workout effort do you suppose is optimal: very easy, easy, moderate, hard, very hard, or all-out?

Let's say, for the sake of discussion, that the optimal effort is the one that feels neither too hard nor too easy, but just right. Which level would be the right effort? Is there, in fact, a single level of workout effort that's optimal for every run? The answer to this question is no, because it's always a mistake to consider the effort of a workout without considering your energy.

It follows that the best answer to the right-effort question is, *it depends on your level of energy.* You are either running too hard, too easy, or just right for the energy of any workout. In order to get workout effort right, you must gauge it to accommodate your workout energy, including both your energy in the moment and the pattern of running energy that develops during the run as a whole.

This means that the apparently simple matter of choosing–the one "right" effort level out of six has been complicated by a factor of five. For six levels of effort and five patterns of energy make a total of thirty effort/energy combinations (see figure 1.3).

Figure 1.3 is a graphic way of illustrating the gamut of effort/energy combinations. The figure is a matrix with 30 cubby-holes, covering the array of combinations from very easy/sluggish (at the bottom left) to all-out/eager (at the top right). This matrix also features five *optimal* workout combinations (those shaded blocks), each of which depends on how much energy you have. For example, when you feel sluggish, the optimal workout effort is very easy. Or when you feel ready-to-run-hard, the optimal workout effort is hard.

	Sluggish	**Tired**	**Lazy**	**Ready**	**Eager**
All-Out	All-Out/ Sluggish	All-Out/ Tired	All-Out/ Lazy	All-Out/ Ready	All-Out/ Eager
Very Hard	Very Hard/ Sluggish	Very Hard/ Tired	Very Hard/ Lazy	Very Hard/ Ready	Very Hard/ Eager
Hard	Hard/ Sluggish	Hard/ Tired	Hard/ Lazy	Hard/ Ready	Hard/ Eager
Moderate	Moderate/ Sluggish	Moderate/ Tired	Moderate/ Lazy	Moderate/ Ready	Moderate/ Eager
Easy	Easy/ Sluggish	Easy/ Tired	Easy/ Lazy	Easy/ Ready	Easy/ Eager
Very Easy	Very Easy/ Sluggish	Very Easy/ Tired	Very Easy/ Lazy	Very Easy/ Ready	Very Easy/ Eager

Figure 1.3 This matrix represents the gamut of effort/energy combinations. Each cube represents a separate workout, consisting of distinct and measurable amounts of effort and energy as defined in this chapter. The optimal combinations are the five shaded ones.

Although effort and energy must both be considered in the adaptive process, energy should be given the primary focus. In practice, you must know how to coordinate your workout efforts with the specific patterns of energy that develop from day to day as you train. Otherwise, your training loses its adaptive focus and you are apt to blunder into over- or undertraining.

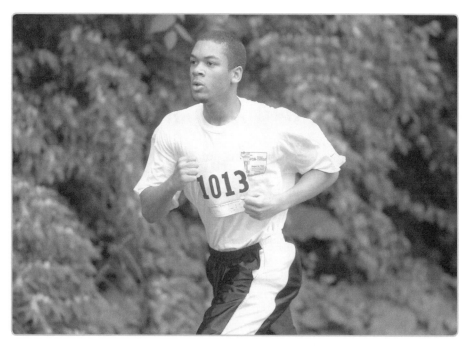

Right effort is running in harmony with your energy, both in the moment and for the workout as a whole.

HARMONIOUS WORKOUTS

The first question I ask myself at the start of every run is, how much energy do I have for this workout? No matter how my energy develops during the whole workout—sluggish, tired, lazy, ready, or eager—the optimal effort will be in harmony with it.

Harmonious workouts are enjoyable, or at least satisfying, rather than burdensome. I look forward to repeating harmonious workouts, rather than being afraid of them because I abhor their difficulty. Harmonious efforts expand my capacity gently during a prolonged warm-up, and they extend the time before fatigue sets in.

An optimal, harmonious workout leaves me feeling as though I could have gone faster or farther than I did. It's tempting to think that I can maximize adaptation by training harder than optimal. Yet, I've learned from experience that disharmonious efforts are not as effective as harmonious workouts because they require reaching beyond my limited capacity for exertion.

Thus, the first question you should ask at the start of every run is, how much energy do I have for this workout? No matter how your energy develops during the workout–sluggish, tired, lazy, ready, or eager–the optimal effort will be in harmony with it.

Your Current Hardest Workout

Your racing ability grows only when you coordinate the effort of your workouts with the energy that develops during them. If you want to become a faster racer you must think in terms of optimizing workout effort to maximize the adaptive value of your workouts.

So far I've used the word "adaptation" without defining it. Here's a practical definition: Adaptation is a long-term increase in your capacity for exertion. Your capacity is your metabolic engine and your gas tank. Adaptation increases your capacity to run longer and/or faster. In this sense, adaptive workouts expand your energy and improve your performance capacity.

At this point, you have in hand the major conceptual constructs of this book. The next step is to use those concepts to understand your capacity for exertion. How does your hardest current workout stack up against the workouts described later in this book? It's crucial that you do an accurate assessment of your hardest workout so you can fit the effort of those new workouts to your current capacity for exertion. Answer the questions in figure 1.4 to determine the hardest workout you currently do on a regular basis.

Your Current Hardest Workout

1. *Workout Effort.* How hard is the workout as a whole?

_____ Very Easy
_____ Easy
_____ Moderate
_____ Hard
_____ Very Hard
_____ All-Out

If these terms are unfamiliar to you, you should review the workout effort scale on pages 7-8.

2. *Level of Fatigue.* How much fatigue do you incur by running this workout?

_____ Imperceptible and insignificant
_____ Perceptible, but negligible
_____ Appreciable, but minor
_____ Noticeable and significant
_____ Obvious and major
_____ Strikingly evident, overwhelming

Are your answers to numbers 1 and 2 consistent? If your hardest workout is a moderate effort, for instance, then your finishing level of fatigue should be close to "appreciable, but minor." See table 1.2 to get an idea of the way these levels of fatigue align themselves with workout effort.

3. *Running Energy.* What are your highest and lowest levels of energy during the workout?

Highest Level:
_____ No energy
_____ Little energy
_____ Some energy
_____ Ample energy
_____ Abundant energy

Lowest Level:
_____ No energy
_____ Little energy
_____ Some energy
_____ Ample energy
_____ Abundant energy

4. *Workout Energy.* What is the pattern of running energy that usually develops during the workout?

_____ Too-*Sluggish*-to-Run-Easy
_____ Too-*Tired*-to-Run-Moderate

(continued)

From *5K and 10K Training* by Brian Clarke, 2006, Champaign, IL: Human Kinetics.

Figure 1.4 (continued)

_____ Too-*Lazy*-to-Run-Hard
_____ *Ready*-to-Run-Hard
_____ *Eager*-to-Race

Are your answers to numbers 3 and 4 consistent? If you say your workout energy is too-tired-to-run-moderate, for instance, then you should have at best little energy during the workout. See the definitions of these terms on pages 10-11.

5. *Effort/Energy Combination.* What are your answers to numbers 1 and 4?

Workout Effort: _____   Workout Energy: _____

Is this workout effort/energy combination optimal, according to figure 1.3 on page 12? If your hardest workout is not an optimal combination, are you overtraining or undertraining according to figure 1.3?

The five questions you just answered focus on the effort and energy of your hardest current workout. Assuming the workout is an optimal effort/energy combination, which of the following combinations comes closest to describing your hardest workout?

Effort/Energy Combination	Capacity
Very Hard/Eager......................	High
Hard/Ready............................	High
Moderate/Lazy........................	Medium
Easy/Lazy..............................	Low
Easy/Tired.............................	Low
Very Easy/Tired.......................	Low
Very Easy/Sluggish..................	Low

Notice the capacity scale in the column on the right. In order to do the workouts described later in this book, you should have at least a medium capacity, as indicated by your hardest current workout. In other words, you should be able to do moderate/lazy workouts. If your workouts have all been easy in recent months, you could still develop the capacity to train at a harder level. But you may need some time to build up to that level without becoming sick, injured, or exhausted by doing something you are not used to doing.

From *5K and 10K Training* by Brian Clarke, 2006, Champaign, IL: Human Kinetics.

Taking the Next Step

An understanding of the ideas in this chapter is crucial to an understanding of the rest of the book. You should see that effort and energy are the fundamental aspects of every run. Similarly, you should understand that effort is made up of two conceptual constructs: workout effort and pace exertion. I defined and delimited these ideas separately and showed you how to use them to think about your training. I also showed you how to think about your running from the perspective of energy, suggesting that energy is made up of two constructs: running energy and workout energy. As you will see throughout this book, energy is the final arbiter in any decision regarding how hard to run.

It's important to realize that you can measure your effort and your energy in the moment or for the workout as a whole. Once you know this, you can think in terms of how you can optimize your effort and energy from moment to moment during a run, as well as for the whole workout. Racing is a special case of effort and energy, because it's beyond normal training levels. In the next chapter, I will raise some issues related to the structure of racing effort and how that structure is affected by your racing energy.

CHAPTER TWO

Structuring Racing Effort

If you are a competitive runner, you are naturally concerned about improving your racing performances. Your ability to perform grows as you adapt to the stress of a series of workouts that simulate some aspect of the race you want to run.

Since you will train with a particular goal-race in mind, you should decide what race you are training for before you begin. This means declaring your intention to run a certain race on a certain date. It also means identifying the specific effort of that race.

I will leave the choice of your goal-race to you. In this chapter, I will describe what I mean by the exertion structure of a goal-race. Once you have a clear idea of that structure, you can design race-specific workouts that will build your ability to run that race effectively.

Estimating Goal-Race Exertion

Your ability-building workouts should be run with a particular goal-race in mind. You should know everything about the race, including its date and distance, its terrain and running surfaces, its possible climatic conditions, and the quality of the competition you might face.

When it comes to training, however, the most important feature of a goal-race is its exertion structure. Each race has a unique and discernable structure, which you can identify by answering two key questions: Approximately how long will it take to finish the race? And what average level of exertion do you want to sustain during that time?

Asking how long you'll need to finish a goal-race is not the same as predicting your fastest possible time. Your time will take care of itself once your training has increased your capacity for exertion. All you need initially is a rough estimate of how long it will take you to finish. That time distinguishes, say, a 5K from a marathon, each of which requires you to race for radically different lengths of time (see figure 2.1).

There are obvious differences in the exertion structures of the races shown in figure 2.1. The heart rate curve for the 5K is relatively short and high, while that of the marathon is relatively long and low. Anyone who has run these racing distances knows that it isn't possible to run a marathon at maximum exertion, because fatigue limits your capacity for exertion.

In general, the higher your average level of exertion during a race, the sooner the onset of fatigue. As you learned in the previous chapter, fatigue increases with the overall effort of a race or workout. So how hard were the races shown in figure 2.1? In fact, the runner rated both races as all-out efforts, meaning he couldn't have run faster for either distance or farther without a crashing slow-down. In this sense, 3 miles at maximum exertion can be just as demanding as 26 miles at steady state. At the finish of both races, this runner was experiencing crushing, inexorable fatigue.

Since both races in figure 2.1 were all-out efforts, it's reasonable to assume that the duration of each race had an impact on the runner's ability to sustain exertion.

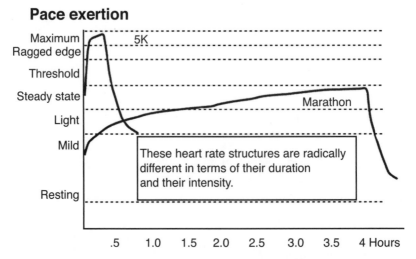

Figure 2.1   These heart rate curves represent two radically different racing structures. First, the 5K took a mere 21 minutes, while the marathon was 11.4 times as long, at 240 minutes. Second, the 5K was run mostly at maximum exertion, while the marathon was run mostly several levels below, at steady state.

It follows that short races can be run at a relatively high level of exertion without a crashing slow-down. And long races must be run at a relatively low level of exertion in order to avoid the same sort of performance-limiting fatigue.

Duration and fatigue have an impact on the level of exertion you are able to sustain in races of different distances. Once you understand how these factors limit your capacity for exertion, you can begin to estimate the maximum level of exertion you'll be able to sustain for a race of any given duration. For the moment, I will assume that you want to run a 10K race in the near future and you are still uncertain how hard you want to exert yourself during the race.

One way to think about your racing effort is to use the components of exertion I described in the first chapter: heart rate, breathing, power, tempo, and intensity. In terms of your breathing, for instance, it's important to know that a very hard 10K goal-race might range from focused but inaudible breathing in the early going, to heavy and audible breathing after the midpoint, and labored breathing from three-quarters until the finish. By contrast, if you want the race to be a hard effort, you might start slower and keep your breathing just under your audible breathing threshold during the second half.

Instead of their racing effort, some runners think of the pace they need to run in order to hit a desired finish time or to beat certain competitors. From this perspective they might become deluded before a big racing event, thinking they can run a pace they simply can't sustain from start to finish. These are usually the athletes who go out too fast and crash well before the finish.

Often their training has given them an inkling of their inability to hold their desired pace, but their ambition blinds them to the realities of their actual performance capacity. Thus, they may overtrain and injure themselves before the race. Or they may suffer anxiety attacks whenever they think about the big event.

The 5K and 10K Racing Effort Continuum

So far, I've skirted around the problem of measuring maximum sustainable exertion. You should see by now that it has to do with the duration of the race you intend to run and the fatigue you can expect to encounter by employing alternate exertion strategies.

But how does talent factor into the exertion equation? Other things being equal, it doesn't matter how talented two runners are. As long as they both run the same duration and the same effort, fatigue limits both to the same maximum sustainable level of exertion (see figure 2.2).

In other words, a jogger and an elite athlete are subject to the same rules that govern pace and exertion. For example, the faster they run during their races, the higher their level of exertion and the sooner fatigue forces itself upon them. If they intend to run all-out for a race as a whole, they must gauge their exertion to bring on just enough fatigue to maintain their average pace to the finish, without crashing.

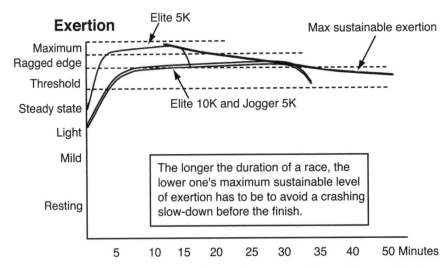

Figure 2.2   The heart rate curves in this graph represent three different all-out races run by a beginning runner and an elite age-group athlete. The elite athlete runs a 5K in less than 15 minutes and, a week later, a 10K in 30 minutes. He runs both races at a maximum sustainable level. Meanwhile, the beginning runner runs an all-out 5K in 30 minutes, also sustaining exertion at her maxim sustainable level. Both 30-minute efforts are virtually identical, albeit for different distances. The maximum sustainable exertion curve shows the average exertion level for an indefinite number of other all-out races in the 13- to 50-minute time frame.

Thus, an elite athlete would run an all-out, 30-minute 10K at the same level of exertion as a less talented runner does an all-out, 30-minute 5K. Furthermore, going out too fast increases their fatigue and destroys their overall performance by forcing a premature and devastating slowdown. On the other hand, going out slower than a maximum sustainable pace gives them a cushion of energy to work with, and may even lead to a more satisfying racing effort.

Structuring Workouts for Maximum Sustainable Exertion

The exertion structure of your workouts depends on the structure of the race you are training for. When your goal-race is the 10K, for instance, the exertion structure of at least some of your workouts should reflect the exertion structure of that race. But how long and how fast should those workouts be? This is one of the fundamental questions of the training process.

Performance Capacity

Planning a new workout for a particular racing distance begins by estimating the level of exertion that will build a desired ability. To illustrate this process, let's

PRERACE WARM-UP

For me, warming up is not about stretching and talking to my friends. I will have stretched at home, and I usually stay away from enjoying the company of friends until after the race. I'm as serious about the warm-up as I am about the race itself, because the quality of the energy and effort I experience in the race will be an extension of the warm-up.

When the gun goes off I want to have saved as much energy as possible for the race itself, and yet I also want to be ready for the exertion a competitive pace will demand of me. The warm-up has to balance these competing goals. Before I start to jog, and depending on the coolness of the morning, I will have stripped down to something light yet heavy enough to enable me to break a sweat with my slowest possible jog.

Remember, I'm not into expending a lot of energy. My attitude can be summed up with a mantra I started using many years ago: I'm calm and in control, and patiently waiting for my body to warm up. I rarely say that mantra anymore because the need to inculcate the attitude it expresses rarely exists. I simply focus on taking short, quick, efficient steps, and feeling for my energy.

I jog so slowly at first that I really can't tell what my energy is like. I've generally given myself about 30 minutes between the start of jogging and the start of the race, so I'll soon find out about my energy. After about 15 or 18 minutes I strip off the remnants of my warm-up clothes and jog in the general direction of the starting line. I still have some things to do, but I want to be in the vicinity of the start so I can feel the energy of the crowd.

Finding a clear stretch of road, I do my first striding pickup for 50 meters. The tempo is between the very slow jog I've been doing and the pace I intend to start the race with in a few minutes. If I've prepared well, I'll be dealing with variations of being eager—somewhere between excellent and superb energy.

The better my energy, the fewer 50-meter strides I'll do. Four is all I ever need to lift my heart rate and get a sense of my starting tempo. It may be the first time in a week or more that I've mustered a racing tempo, but all I need is a gentle reminder. Then I dive into the crowd of runners, ideally with less than a minute or two before the gun, and seek out my racing peers.

study the case of a 30-year-old male runner named John who wants to build his speed and endurance for a 10K.

What sort of workout can John employ that would enable him to practice speed and endurance? Let's say that speed is John's ability to outsprint a competitor at the finish of a race, and endurance is his ability to sustain the specific discomfort of his 10K race. For the moment, let's also say that speed and endurance for the 10K are related to John's audible breathing threshold.

RACING VERY HARD/EAGER

Over the years, I've honed my outlook to a point where racing very hard/eager is a given. I may think about how to perform in a race, but I don't worry about my ability to perform. I simply go out and perform. And, provided I run very hard/eager, I know my performance will take care of itself. It may not be good enough to win in every case, but I will perform to my credit.

Sometimes, when my energy is as good as it gets and the competition is also there, I might decide to run all-out/eager. But I never go into a race intending to run all-out because I'm never sure that circumstances will favor all-out racing. Racing all-out/eager can be extremely difficult and dissonant. By contrast, very hard/eager is harmonious and exhilarating. So I aim for the mentally acceptable racing level, and I deal with unforeseeable circumstances as they arise in the defining moment of a race.

Every race has its defining competitive moment. It's the point where I must respond to a challenge or lose the race. Often, circumstances call for a creative response on my part. As a competitive athlete I have to find a way to win, whether by surging away or perhaps by following at a distance.

During the first half of many 10K races, I've deliberately fallen back, not knowing whether I could reel the competition in during the second half. Yet rarely have I lost a race like that, because I know I can beat anyone of my ability who goes out too fast.

When John first started doing 10Ks with a heart rate monitor, he was surprised to find his audible breathing threshold was about 88 percent of his maximum heart rate. Typically, his audible breathing threshold had been about 80 percent of maximum during his hard workouts. In other words, his audible-breathing threshold was about 8 percent lower in training than it was in a race. If training for speed and endurance is related to John's audible breathing threshold, which heart rate level would be most relevant in the training context: 80 percent or 88 percent of maximum?

In answering this question for yourself, keep in mind that your heart rate is tied up with your experience of running energy. Having abundant energy–as you might during a race–enables you to run at a faster pace for a longer time than you could when you have only ample energy, as you would during a hard workout. Since your heart rate is keyed by your pacing, the faster you run the higher your heart rate rises. It follows that your heart rate will be higher in a race than in most training runs primarily because your pace is faster, but also because your racing energy is typically better than your training energy.

This extra racing energy distorts your experience of race exertion. With regard to the power component of exertion, for instance, you feel light as a feather and relaxed at a racing pace and heart rate that you might be able to achieve only by pressing the pace during most training runs. Similarly, as we've seen in John's case, you might begin to hear your breathing at about 80 percent of maximum during training, where you might begin to hear it at close to 90 percent of maximum during a race. The figures in this example may not be exactly the same for you personally; in general, though, racing heart rate is significantly higher than training heart rate, especially when your energy is substantially better, too.

In other words, performance capacity is ordinarily greater during a race than a workout. This is particularly true when your workouts are scheduled so close to one another that you don't have a chance to recover fully from them as you would for a race. When you have less than top energy, your capacity alters the texture of exertion, slowing you down and making a run seem more difficult.

Racing Energy and the Workout Planning Process

Let's return to the example of our 30-year-old male athlete named John. The lower levels of energy John experiences in training will affect the heart rate structure of the workout he is planning. For instance, when it comes to structuring exertion to build endurance, his workout pace will be slower than his race pace because he has less energy for the workout. Thus, in general, one can simulate the specific exertion of any race at a lower training heart rate than the race itself.

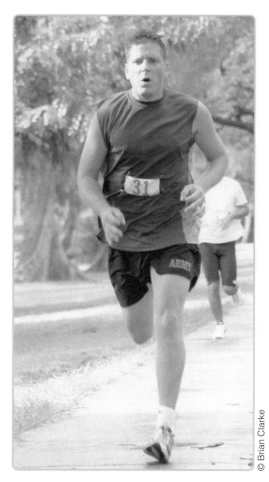

Take a look at figure 2.3 on page 26, which illustrates this principle. There, I've juxtaposed the heart rate structures of John's endurance/speed workout and his 10K race. Notice that the workout heart rate curve in figure 2.3 is lower than the race, yet that workout structure is in the same relative position as John's audible-breathing threshold during the race.

Remember, you will usually have more energy for a race than a workout. Since your energy influences your perception of exertion, you can simulate specific aspects of your race without actually running at race pace or having your heart rate at the racing level. Thus, when you first start doing a workout, it's better to focus on perceived exertion than to focus on a predetermined racing pace.

Being eager to race gives you abundant energy and an aggressive attitude, both of which are necessary to exert a competitive effort.

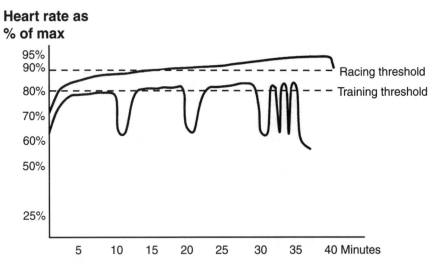

Figure 2.3   This graph shows the heart rate curves of a Very Hard/Eager 10K race (the top curve) in relation to a Hard/Ready workout (the warm-up jogs are not shown). The workout curve is lower than the racing curve because the runner's energy for the workout was less than his energy for the race. Nonetheless, workout exertion is specific to race exertion because, in both cases, the runner's heart rate is in the same relative position to his audible breathing threshold.

When you become pace-obsessed during training, you'll almost always run too fast for your training energy. As a coach, I've discovered this to be a difficult idea to sell to a group of inexperienced but ambitious runners who are focused mainly on their pace. There is usually a chorus of concern expressed whenever I order them to practice their racing tempo at a pace that's the same or slower than their racing pace. How—they want to know—can they get faster if they don't train faster than they race? My answer: Pace is not the primary adaptive stimulus.

Exertion is the primary adaptive stimulus. When it comes to practicing the specific exertion of the race you want to run, you must think in terms of how that exertion feels. When it comes to the tempo and power components of exertion, for instance, does the race feel slow and comfortable, quick and relaxed, rapid and pressed or fast and forced? In other words, how can you simulate the feeling of a race during a workout?

Once you have an accurate heart rate record and a good mental picture of the race you want to run, you'll have a much clearer idea of the training necessary to prepare for the race. The art of planning a new workout is to structure it in relation to your goal-event. A relatively long, slow race like a marathon will require relatively longer, slower training runs than those required for a 5K.

All-Out/Eager Races

Racing efforts are competitive. Unless you prefer to finish and enjoy your races, your intention will be to compete and perform in them. You won't necessarily care about being the overall winner, but you'll know who your competitors are and you'll want to perform well enough to beat them, which could mean running very hard or all-out.

Training efforts, by contrast, occupy the lower effort levels, according to your energy. The more energy you have the harder you may train. But hard workouts are generally the hardest efforts you should attempt in training because workouts, by definition, are noncompetitive. Their only purpose is to build racing ability. If you are racing people in your workouts, you may be having fun but you aren't proving a thing.

You cannot establish racing dominance by beating someone in a workout. Racing a workout is like sneaking up on someone and hitting them from behind, especially when you take the opportunity to race a workout only when you are feeling eager-to-race. If your training partner is only ready-to-run-hard, as he should be for a hard workout, you claim a hollow victory when you "beat" him because he wasn't at his best in terms of energy. The expectations for a race are different than those for a workout. When you put yourself on the line for a race, you declare that you're at your best and you're willing to race anyone of your ability who stands with you on that line.

You don't need to train very hard or all-out in order to improve. When it comes to head-to-head racing, however, very hard and all-out efforts are the norm. The object is to beat your competitors, and if they are running very hard you have to run a comparable effort, too. I realize, of course, that many people are not so competitively inclined. Most of the recreational runners and joggers in my training programs, for instance, run moderate-to-hard races, demonstrating their predilection to finish and enjoy them rather than compete and perform in them.

As they gain experience in the racing game, some of these athletes become increasingly competitive–if only to compete with themselves for faster finishing times. They are generally the sort of people who are concerned about their performance in other parts of their life, as well. Since achieving a time is closely associated with effort, they gradually intensify their racing efforts as their ambition grows. In the process, they soon conclude that the quality of a racing performance depends on energy as much as effort.

The size of an effort and the performance it generates are directly related to your capacity for exertion. Having abundant energy, for instance, makes an all-out effort huge, which makes its performance relatively fast, too. Figure 2.4 illustrates this point by comparing a hard/ready workout with an all-out/eager race.

You can't run harder than your capacity allows. Of course, once you've run all-out, you can continue running–albeit at a much slower pace. You can even drive yourself into extreme fatigue, with your body producing energy inefficiently from fat and muscle protein. But this sort of exhaustive running is outside of normal training and racing. The size of an effort depends on your capacity, and being eager-to-race provides the largest capacity.

Thus, the primary problem is to start a race at the eager level. Peaking, tapering, and carbohydrate loading are important aspects of a solution to this problem. Having effective pre-race routines and knowing how to focus your attention are two other important aspects of the competitive game.

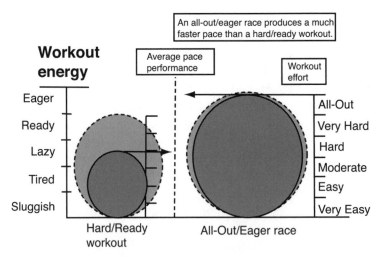

Figure 2.4 You cannot run harder than your energy allows, which explains why both workout effort scales are the same height as the capacity circles. Since eager is greater than ready, and all-out is greater than hard, it follows that an all-out/eager racing effort is much greater than a hard/ready workout effort. Since average pace "rides on a wheel of effort," the race pace in this example is faster than the training pace.

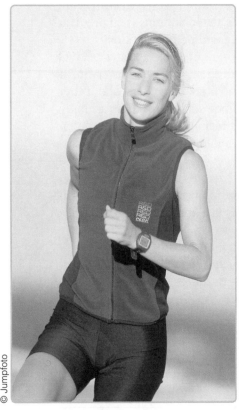

Setting Up Your Goal-Race

Before you consider issues related to establishing new ability-building workouts, you should choose the goal-race for which those workouts will prepare you. How long will the race be and how hard do you plan to run it?

Because elite athletes run at a faster pace than joggers, they will structure the exertion of their 5K or 10K races differently from jogger-athletes running the same distance. By answering the questions in figure 2.5 you will be better able to understand the structure of your particular goal-race.

The way you train will be the way you race. Thus, harmonious training leads to harmonious racing.

Figure 2.5
Structuring Your Goal-Race

1. *Approximate Race Duration.* How long will the race take you to finish?

> Time in minutes: _____
> Distance of event: _____
> Pace in minutes per mile: _____

The faster you can run in minutes per mile, the better your performance capacity. Running under five minutes a mile for 5K or 10K, for instance, would put you in the elite category when it comes to estimating your capacity to perform.

But other factors will determine your actual level of exertion, including the duration of your event, your willingness to suffer intense discomfort, and your susceptibility to injury.

2. *Racing Orientation.* One of the key factors in determining your racing effort is your competitive orientation, whether you mostly want to finish and enjoy your goal-race or whether you want to compete and perform in it. Where do you stand on the following scale?

> Finish/Enjoy   1-----2-----3-----4-----5   Compete/Perform

Although both orientations tend to overlap, your particular orientation will determine the overall effort of your race and, to some extent, the overall effort of your workouts.

3. *Overall Effort.* How hard will your goal-race be? The following scale answers this question in terms of how you will feel at the finish.

> > **Moderate:** Still very energetic in the last mile, and only somewhat fatigued at the finish. A low-risk effort, but not very satisfying. Nowhere near a fastest performance.
> > **Hard:** Noticeably fatigued, but capable of blasting the pace in the last mile. A good and satisfying effort, but not close to your fastest possible performance.
> > **Very Hard:** Very fatigued at the finish, but capable of going on a while longer without crashing. Capable of mustering a sprint to the finish. Close to your fastest possible performance.
> > **All-Out:** Barely maintaining your pace at finish; couldn't go on without a crashing slowdown. Couldn't run faster for the race as a whole.

(continued)

Figure 2.5 *(continued)*

Your racing orientation, as described in the previous question, will influence your answer to this question. A strong compete/perform orientation, for example, will facilitate your willingness to run a racing effort with greater intensity.

Athletes who are mostly oriented toward finishing and enjoying, as well as those who are at risk for injury, might want to aim for a moderate-to-hard effort initially. Ambitious athletes and people who want to test themselves at an intense level can start with a very hard racing effort.

Unless your energy and the competitive circumstances of a particular race lend themselves to running all-out, I don't recommend intentionally planning to run all-out races. It's like playing poker. You wouldn't decide to go all-in before you see how a hand develops.

4. *Average Level of Exertion.* What average level of exertion will you sustain during the race?

> **Mild:** Your slowest jogging pace. Gentle and soothing.
> **Light:** A conversational tempo, holding back the pace. Very comfortable.
> **Steady state:** A relaxed tempo, with deep, slow, inaudible breathing and a "huff" between phrases of conversation. Still comfortable.
> **Threshold:** A pressed tempo, with audible, controlled, but heavy breathing.
> **Ragged edge:** A forced tempo with labored, noisy breathing after the midpoint. Uncomfortable.
> **Maximum:** A strained tempo after the midpoint, with labored/hyperfast breathing. Very uncomfortable.

The harder your overall effort, the closer you'll have to run to your maximum sustainable level of exertion for the race as a whole. If you aren't sure about your maximum sustainable exertion level, you might want to run a practice race, going out at steady state and gradually increasing your exertion until you develop a sense of your max for a particular racing distance.

Once you have a good mental picture of the race you want to run, you'll have a much clearer idea of the training necessary to prepare for it. The art of planning a new workout is to structure it in relation to your goal-event. The shorter the race the shorter your race-specific workouts need to be.

From *5K and 10K Training* by Brian Clarke, 2006, Champaign, IL: Human Kinetics.

Taking the Next Step

In this chapter I've presented ways to gauge the effort of a goal-race. Understanding your racing effort begins with an understanding of how hard you will run from moment to moment during the run, which in turn determines the overall effort of the race. A race is generally different from a training run because it requires harder effort and greater energy. Except for a few suggestions in the sidebar on page 38, I'm not concerned in this book with how to gather your energy for a race. Rather, I want you to know how to structure your exertion so you achieve your competitive goals without hurting your performance by going out too fast and becoming prematurely fatigued.

Once you know the exertion structure of the race you intend to run, you have a basis for planning workouts that will prepare you specifically for that race. Any workout has the potential to build five distinct abilities: stamina, power, tempo, speed, and endurance. The next chapter will focus on how to distinguish between these abilities so you can structure workouts to build them.

CHAPTER 3

Practicing the Five Racing Abilities

The process of planning a new workout always begins with consideration of your ability-building purpose. Since the ultimate purpose of competitive training is to make you a faster racer, all workouts should support this purpose. I realize this competitive view of training disregards other reasons for working out, such as releasing stress or simply enjoying a run. Nonetheless, if your primary reason for training is to prepare for a race, then other reasons must take a backseat to your competitive purpose. Ultimately, that purpose will be to build your racing ability.

Racing ability is the capacity to exert yourself exactly as you want in a particular race. You should have at least enough stamina to cover the distance without stopping, enough muscle power to run relaxed at your racing pace, enough tempo ability to run comfortably at that pace, enough endurance to sustain the pace against the onslaught of second-half fatigue, and enough speed to outsprint your competition at the finish.

Everyone has these five racing abilities in at least some small measure. The goal of training is to become fully capable of using each ability in a race, and the only way you can build an ability is by practicing it in training. So which of the five abilities do you want to practice? And how will you structure the exertion of your workouts to practice those abilities?

The first part of this chapter will give you a conceptual understanding of the five racing abilities, and the next part will further your understanding so you can target race-specific levels of exertion to achieve your particular ability-building purpose.

The Five Racing Abilities

The concepts that delimit the five racing abilities are marked by several essential ideas. The following material will show how the five abilities differ from one another so you can understand their distinctions.

At first glance, for instance, stamina and endurance may seem like indistinguishable ideas, but they are entirely different concepts in the system I'm describing. Stamina is the ability to run long and slow, while endurance is the ability to sustain uncomfortable race exertion. These definitions have drastic implications for the way you would structure your workouts to build each ability.

Long, Slow Runs Build Stamina

The essential ingredient of a stamina workout is slow running, meaning light exertion. Light exertion is marked by inaudible, conversational breathing at 60 to 69 percent of your maximum heart rate. You have to hold yourself back to train for stamina. It's okay to run even slower, at mild exertion, as you warm up or when you are too tired during recovery runs to maintain light exertion. But, for our purposes, steady state is too quick for long duration.

The goal of stamina training is to increase your ability to run long and slow. Increased stamina shows up as the ability to do progressively longer workouts at light exertion. If you are building weekly mileage, the goal is to add duration to all or some of your workouts while maintaining adequate energy for each workout. In other words, workout duration grows because adaptation increases your capacity for long, slow running.

You aren't building stamina unless you can run progressively longer workouts at light exertion with the same amount of running energy. In this process, your pace is immaterial because all that matters is the duration of light-exertion running.

© Jumpfoto

The essential ingredient of a stamina workout is slow, light-exertion running at a conversational breathing level.

Long, Intense Repetitions Build Endurance

If stamina is the ability to run long and slow, what is endurance? According to the way I'm defining the term, endurance is the ability to sustain race pace at an uncomfortable level of exertion.

Because any racing distance can be uncomfortable, it follows that all races demand endurance—even relatively short races like the 5K or 10K. Short races can cause as much discomfort as a marathon, albeit for a much shorter timeframe. In order to build endurance, you have to structure workouts that demand race-specific amounts of discomfort. This is different from stamina training, which restricts you by definition to a very comfortable level of exertion.

Whether you are training for a mile or a marathon, endurance workouts are tough to do because the duration of the tempo effort is long enough to simulate the specific discomfort of the second half of a race, when fatigue becomes a major factor. A lot of the discomfort of a race near the finish is due to extreme fatigue. An endurance workout doesn't have this extreme fatigue because it is typically only a noticeably fatiguing, hard workout—not an all-out race. The exertion of an endurance workout should feel like the exertion in the middle to late stages of your goal-race, minus the extreme fatigue.

Although endurance workouts incorporate an element of intensity, they can't be so intense that the workout effort exceeds your adaptive limit. Typically, this means the workout should be short enough to qualify as hard, rather than very hard. It also means inserting rest intervals to break up race-specific tempo running into several repetitions. Each rest interval should be long and slow enough that you are able to start the next tempo repetition at least somewhat refreshed.

This view of endurance training is different from the common idea of long, slow runs that build endurance. Remember, stamina and endurance are different abilities, requiring different sorts of exertion structures. Nonetheless, a long, slow run can take on the marks of an endurance workout when it is so long that heavy fatigue causes you to encounter uncomfortable exertion before the finish.

If your stamina workouts feel like endurance workouts, you are probably running too long for your adaptive purpose. You must be clear about your purpose, and structure your stamina and endurance workouts accordingly.

Pace-Specific Intervals Build Racing Tempo

Tempo and speed are also different abilities, with different definitions. Tempo is the ability to run comfortably at race pace, while speed is the ability to surge for a short distance at a pace that's faster than your average race pace.

Tempo training is important because—more than speed work—it determines how fast you'll be able to run the race. If you want to race at a quick tempo, for instance, you've got to practice a quick tempo. It's that simple. Moreover, you've got to be able to maintain that tempo without running into major fatigue and discomfort during the first half of the race. It takes a lot of tempo training to build an adequate base of tempo ability.

Tempo workouts, like their endurance counterparts, are built on the specific tempo of your goal-race, whether fast or slow. But, unlike endurance training, where the object is to simulate the specific discomfort of the second half of a race, tempo training simulates the specific comfort of the first half. Since your particular racing tempo could be fast, obviously you won't be able to maintain that tempo in training for very long and have it still be comfortable. The trick in avoiding discomfort, therefore, is to run short tempo intervals with frequent rests.

Tempo training is usually intervallic, meaning you repeat many bouts of tempo running within a single workout. There are two sorts of intervals: tempo intervals and rest intervals. Intermittent rest-jogs, lasting about a minute to 90 seconds (depending on the length of the tempo interval), should bring your heart rate down at least one full exertion level. These regular drops in exertion keep your tempo running from becoming as intense as it can be during an endurance workout in which you employ the same tempo with less frequent rest breaks.

To train at racing tempo is not necessarily to train at racing pace, but at a pace that feels like race pace. Your actual workout pace (measured in minutes per mile) will usually be between race pace and about 10 percent slower, depending on your energy. Since it's difficult to run at racing tempo without sufficient energy, I don't recommend running that fast in training unless your running energy is at least ample, as it should be for a hard workout. You have to pick your moments to do pace-specific tempo training, confining it to planned workouts when you have sufficient energy. Otherwise, if you do intervals with less than ample energy, they must be short enough and slow enough to accommodate whatever energy you have.

This is not the same as running out of energy in a race. Late in a race, you may have to force the pace to counter the effects of fatigue. But forcing your pace is not the experience we are trying to simulate in tempo training. Rather, you should simulate your racing tempo during the first half of a race when your energy is still good and you can pound along feeling relaxed at race pace.

Interval workouts should be carefully designed to achieve a particular ability-building purpose. If your tempo intervals are too short, you'll tend to run them at a pace that's faster than your current race pace, which makes them by definition speed work, not tempo training. On the other hand, if the intervals are too long, they will become uncomfortable at your current racing tempo, which makes them endurance repetitions, not tempo intervals.

Up-Tempo Repetitions Build Speed

Speed is completely different from tempo. You don't have speed unless you can accelerate above your average race pace when you are fatigued, and when anaerobic acidosis is a major deterrent to your ability to beat a close competitor.

While some people make a show of flying at the finish of a race, their speed only indicates that they could have run faster for the race as a whole. Speed exists when you've run at least a very hard racing effort, and yet you can still muster a faster-than-average pace to surge away at a crucial juncture or outsprint a competitor in the final moments. With the finish line in sight, a final sprint will have little impact on your average pace for the whole distance, but it could mean the difference between winning and losing.

Speed work in the training context is not usually maximum-effort sprinting. Rather, it should bear some relation to the pace and distance of the actual sprint you might have to sustain to beat someone in a race. Remember, your top speed at the end of a race when you are fatigued is not the same as your top speed when you are fresh and rested. In structuring speed work, the first question is, what faster-than-average pace can you reasonably expect to achieve? I think of it as a notch up from racing tempo, say, from quick to rapid or from rapid to fast.

Moreover, you must ask yourself how far you can reasonably expect to hold a finishing kick. Since you can't expect to sprint for your entire racing distance, you likewise don't need a lot of speed work to be prepared to sprint at the finish. It's usually sufficient to tack on a little speed work at the end of a tempo or endurance workout when you are already warmed up for tempo running, and you can safely increase your pace a notch above your maximum sustainable racing tempo (see figure 2.3 on page 26 for an example of this sort of workout).

It's important to ask yourself during a tempo workout whether you could hold that tempo for your entire racing distance. If you feel you can't, you aren't building tempo, but speed. Many runners believe they have to train faster than their current race pace to become a faster racer. I don't dispute their logic; rather, I

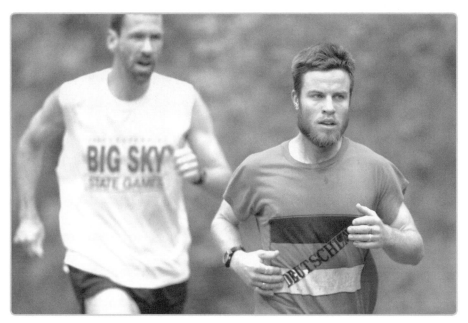

Speed work is not maximum effort sprinting, but it can be intensely focused and a notch up from racing tempo.

EAGER TO RACE

Suppose you had to declare your intention before every race. What would you intend for yourself? At a minimum, I would want to be eager-to-race so I would have the energy to accomplish whatever additional goals I might have. My declaration to be eager would also establish my commitment to be on top of my game for the race.

There is a lot of power in the act of declaration. It's the power to alter your physical status or shift your way of being. Declaring something about a race assumes you've envisioned a set of conditions for yourself. Without envisioning these conditions you couldn't bring them into being. So that's the first step. Next you have to enter into a conversation with yourself about meeting those conditions. In this case, the issue is how to greatly expand your performance capacity on the day of an event.

At the most mundane level, you'll need a plan for gathering your energy. That includes tapering your training, eating and resting well, and focusing your intent. Since you won't always be in the midst of a peaking schedule when you decide to race, you won't necessarily have a lot of energy available for racing. During base-building or sharpening periods, for instance, your energy will usually be lazy or ready, but rarely eager. So it will take a commitment on your part to do whatever is necessary to increase your energy beyond its usual level.

Aside from adequate rest, carbohydrate loading is the most effective way to increase your energy for a race. You may think that you eat plenty of starchy foods, but do you eat pasta morning, noon, and night in the last few days before a race? You may think that the 5K or 10K distance is too short to bother about carbo loading. But if you want to feel and perform your best, then you may have to take radical measures to suffuse your leg muscles with glycogen.

Pasta is better than rice, and rice is better than potatoes for carbo loading. But I've known runners who fill a plate with potatoes, rice *and* pasta 36 hours before a race knowing that food will be where they want it the morning of the race.

offer a different point of view. First, training faster than race pace limits workout duration, and it's the *duration* of tempo training that builds the capacity to sustain your pace for the full duration of a race.

Second, pace is not the adaptive stimulus for improving your capacity; it's exertion at your racing tempo that stimulates adaptive processes. Have faith. As long as your training pace improves with adaptation, your racing pace will improve as well.

Resistance Training Builds Power

Power and tempo are closely related abilities. Tempo is the ability to run *comfortably* at race pace, while power is the ability to run *relaxed* at race pace. Tempo is about sustaining a specific rate of motion; power is about covering ground with each stride.

Do you realize that when two athletes run a mile at the same quick, relaxed tempo, they both run the same number of steps per minute? The more powerful of the two, however, might run the mile in six minutes while the weaker does it in eight minutes. They both run at the same quick tempo but the stronger runner takes longer strides.

Similarly, when the same two athletes run a six-minute mile, the stronger runner will still run at a quick, relaxed, steady-state level. But the other athlete keeps up only by forcing his pace at ragged-edge exertion. The weaker runner takes more steps during his six-minute mile because he is running at his fastest sustainable tempo. Meanwhile, the stronger runner could move away from the slower runner by simply lengthening and quickening his stride.

Natural ability is a function of individual talent. The most talented runners are innately faster than the least talented. Nonetheless, anyone can build beyond his or her natural endowment with adaptive training. So how do you become a stronger, more powerful runner? In recent years, we've learned to build power with biking, weightlifting, stair climbing, and plyometrics. But the traditional way to build muscle strength for running is with hill work.

Running Hills

You have to make clear distinctions between running on the flats and in the hills. Since I am not a kinesiologist, I can't explain all the biomechanical differences. I do know, however, that running in the hills changes my running form, compared to running on flat surfaces. An uphill grade forces me to lower my chin and lean forward slightly in order to shift my center of gravity toward the balls of my feet. The steeper the hill, the more pronounced these changes, all of which place markedly increased stress on my feet, Achilles tendons, and calf muscles. These are the same structures that help to move my body ahead over the ground. So naturally, they stand to gain from the added stress of hill work.

Hill work does build muscle strength for running. But it is also potentially injurious. The same stress that leads to adaptation in the hills can also lead to injured metatarsals, Achilles tendons, and calf muscles. Heavy people who are out of shape have to be especially careful in the hills because their size puts an added burden on these physical structures. The underlying problem, though, has to do with the way we think about our hill work. Our false attitudes and misconceptions can lead us into major blunders, which can easily take us out of the game until we've recovered. Probably the most prevalent mistake I've witnessed in my years as a coach and runner is the tendency to run too fast in the hills.

The first rule of successful hill running is to slow down whenever you encounter a hill. You can continue running at your racing tempo, but your stride length has to be shorter than it would be on level ground. Of course, a shorter stride means a slower pace but it also means you can keep your exertion within targeted, adaptive bounds. The steeper the hill, the more you have to slow down in order to maintain the right level of exertion and the proper level of resistance.

Remember, too much resistance is downright inefficient. It also increases your risk of injury. So the question is, how much resistance is enough to build your muscle strength for a particular goal-race?

For training purposes, the most logical level of resistance is the specific level encountered in your goal-race. It follows that relatively long, slow, steady-state hill work is appropriate for a marathoner, while shorter, steeper hills at higher levels of exertion are more appropriate for a miler. That said, the caveat to the general resistance training mandate is this: You must be sufficiently in shape to survive the specific level of resistance demanded by your goal-race. It could, for instance, take several cycles of marathon-like training in the hills before you are ready to power up at levels called for by a relatively short racing distance.

One guideline for building power in the hills is to stay relaxed, no matter how hard your particular regimen requires you to work. This principle may sound paradoxical when you are training for a short race that requires you to press or force the pace. But remember, you are trying to build enough power to run relaxed during the first half of your race. If you constantly press the pace in training, you won't learn to run relaxed. Again, the trick is to structure hill (or tempo) intervals that are short enough so you finish relaxed, regardless of your pace. The moment you are about to press, it's time to slow down and take a rest.

A final guideline for building power in the hills is to maintain your running form: chin down, elbows back, arms relaxed. Your head shouldn't stick out in front of you, but simply tilt forward with a lowered chin. Correct form on a hill is mostly about balancing your body on the smaller platform of the forward part of your feet. Your upper body should be erect above your hips without the feeling of being tilted backward. Your whole body should have enough tilt from the level of your feet that you sense some forward momentum. Doing this correctly on a steep hill requires getting up on the balls of your feet and springing off the ground from your ankles using the strength of your calves.

Few people have the strength to run up steep hills on the balls of their feet, especially at a race-specific level. The better way is to slow down initially and strive for correct form in the hills. Your visual focus should be on the ground a few meters in front of you, not on the top of the hill. If you aren't strong enough to get off your heels completely, try having them kiss the ground and lift off lightly. To do this with proper form, you'll need a hill with a forgiving grade. In other words, don't start hill training with the steepest hill in town. Look for gentle hills that allow you to maintain your form while you learn to stress your feet and calves. Add hills in small doses to your long runs or easy workouts and take a long-range view to building power. The steepest hills will still be there a couple years from now.

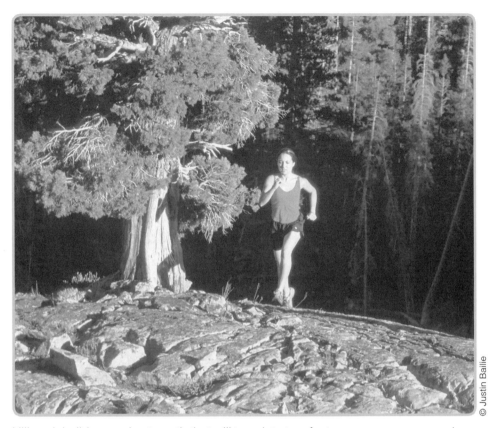

© Justin Bailie

Hill work builds muscle strength that will translate to a faster race pace on race day.

Setting Up Workouts to Build Ability

The foregoing material should have given you a conceptual understanding of the five racing abilities. In order to apply these concepts to your training, you'll need to know how to set up a new workout. Setting up a workout is the process of planning, designing, and establishing a workout as a viable, adaptive entity.

The planning and design stage should occur before you take a running step. You must have an idea of the ability you aim to build and the workout structure that will achieve that purpose in relation to a goal-race. I realize that thinking about a new workout isn't as much fun as actually running it. But, unless you choose to follow someone else's workouts for the rest of your running career, you must be able to envision effective workouts before you run them.

Once envisioned, establishing a workout is what you do when you actually run a new workout the first few times. It isn't easy to get it right the first time out. If you've scheduled the workout inappropriately, or if your design is faulty, the workout will most likely result in injury or illness instead of improved ability. Ultimately, you have to establish the exertion structure of the workout as an adaptive stimulus before you can gain adaptive value from it.

You can build ability only by repeating an established workout during a training period. But the setup process is a hurdle you have to negotiate before the ability-building process can begin. Thus, setting up a workout is one of the major, recurrent problems of the overall training process. Every time you begin a new training period, you must solve the setup problem.

Target Zones and Heart Rate Limits

Since setting up a new workout is such an integral part of training, I will develop the topic in several parts of this book. Here, as a way of introducing the problem in context with the theme of purposeful workouts, I will introduce the case of a 30-year-old female athlete named Tanya.

The problem I gave Tanya when she first started training under my tutelage was to establish a 40-minute recovery run that would leave enough energy for the two hard workouts on her weekly schedule. As long as she had sufficient energy for her hard workouts, she could run the easy workout as many times as she wanted, up to twice a day. It took her about a month to settle into a workout regimen that included the two hard workouts, plus seven easy recovery runs a week. Figure 3.1 is the graph of one of those easy 40-minute runs.

Figure 3.1 shows that Tanya's heart rate rose through her mild- and light-exertion levels during the easy workout. (Note: I've evened out minor ups and downs related to hills and other pacing anomalies, as I have with every heart rate

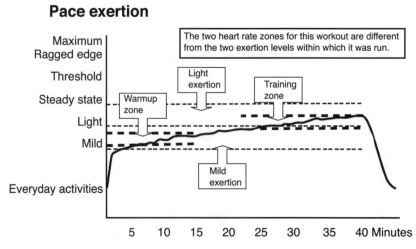

Figure 3.1 This graph illustrates the distinction between exertion levels and target zones. The heart rate curve rose between the mild and light exertion levels during this 40-minute workout. It also rose through two target zones, the purposes of which were to guide the runner through the warm-up portion of her run, and through the subsequent training portion.

curve in this book.) Tanya's heart rate curve only hints at how she established this particular workout. Why is it that she began the workout at mild exertion? Why does she finish at mid-light exertion? Why doesn't her heart rate seem to level out at a target rate? Did she even have a target heart rate?

In order to answer these questions we should agree that a target heart rate is different from an exertion level. An exertion level is delimited by characteristics that make it distinct from adjoining levels. For example, light exertion is distinct from mild exertion in that mild exertion represents one's slowest jogging pace while light exertion can be faster as long as it doesn't exceed conversational breathing and 69 percent of maximum heart rate. A target heart rate, by contrast, is the specific heart rate needed to accomplish a training purpose, such as building a racing ability or recovering from a prior workout. In this sense, target heart rates guide a runner to structure a workout with a purpose.

Tanya's ability-building purpose was to do some stamina training during recovery periods between hard workouts. Since she had to be recovered to do her hard workouts in certain weekly time slots, her recovery runs had to be easy enough to maintain adequate energy in those time slots. In this regard, there is no substitute for the trial and error process of actually doing a workout to see whether it achieves your purpose. Thus, before Tanya could declare a target heart rate, she had to discover a heart rate progression for the workout that would enable her to accomplish her recovery purpose.

Tanya started by repeating the easy workout several times a week to see how it would feel in relation to the hard workouts on her schedule. She noticed immediately that, during her recovery runs, she was often tired from the hard workouts, which meant that she had little energy at the start of the easy workout and didn't feel like running fast. In fact, she had to jog very slowly while she warmed up to keep her effort from being injurious and burdensome.

She also noticed that when she pressed above a certain heart rate during the warm-up she tended to run out of energy before the end of the recovery run. This negatively affected her energy for her next hard workout. Similarly, she noticed that when she went above a certain heart rate at the end of the recovery run—when her energy was finally turning on—she didn't have enough energy for the next hard workout.

Because her primary objective was to run easy enough that she could recover for her next hard workout, she decided to set heart rate limits above which she couldn't go if she wanted to achieve her objective. Thus, she developed two target zones based on her experience of doing the workout: one for the warm-up and the other for the second portion of the workout when her energy was better.

Tanya's energy was the key to optimizing the effort of this recovery run. As a coach, I couldn't determine how much energy she would have for any given workout. Thus, I couldn't tell her exactly how hard to run. All runners have to adjust their effort according to their energy. This central optimizing principle applies to all workouts, whether you want them to be hard or easy.

Being Clear About Your Purpose

There are five racing abilities and, therefore, five ability-building purposes. Each purpose should result in a unique workout structure but the pace-specific abilities—tempo and endurance—actually employ the specific tempo of your goal-race. Let's consider the process of setting up a tempo workout.

Given the goal of racing a 10K, your training tempo should feel slower than it would if you were training for a 5K. I'm not saying you shouldn't train at 5K tempo when training for a 10K. I'm simply pointing out that when you aim to simulate 10K tempo in a workout there's a clear distinction between that tempo and the one you would hold for a shorter, faster race. We have to make choices about where we will apply our energy, as we can't prepare effectively for the gamut of racing distances all at once.

Depending on your natural talent, 10K tempo will feel quick and relaxed or rapid and pressed, but probably not fast and forced. This is something you may have to think about the next time you run a 10K. How does the tempo feel? How many steps are you taking per minute? How many steps per minute are optimal in terms of efficient pace performance? Remember, the most talented runners finish the 10K in fewer than 30 minutes, while many others finish closer to 60 minutes. The shorter duration of an elite runner's race can make it possible to press the pace, while the longer duration of a slower runner's race requires a more relaxed pace.

In addition to the specific tempo of the race you aim to run, you should also consider your target heart rate. In order to zero in on the heart rate of various ability-building workouts, you might try graphing your training heart rate in relation to your racing heart rate. The higher your average goal-race heart rate, the higher your average workout heart rate should be, without actually reaching the racing level (see figure 3.2).

Notice from figure 3.2 that there is little to distinguish hill work from tempo work when it comes to targeting training heart rate. During both sorts of workouts—whether on the flats or in the hills—you should aim your heart rate for the middle ground between light exertion and the maximum sustainable exertion for your racing distance.

The higher your maximum sustainable racing heart rate for a specific racing distance, the higher your training heart rate should be to build muscle strength and tempo for that distance. When training in the hills, however, you must also make distinctions between pace, tempo, and heart rate. You can maintain your racing tempo in the hills, for instance, but you must take shorter steps, which makes for a slower pace and a more appropriate training heart rate.

As you can see, right exertion depends on the way you coordinate a number of variables. These include your individual talent, your chosen goal-race, your current racing pace, your ability-building purpose, and your training heart rate. Given the complexity of the setup process, you must assume major responsibility for setting up your own right exertion workouts.

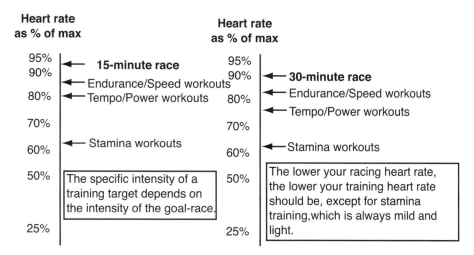

Figure 3.2   This graph illustrates training targets in preparation for a 15-minute race and a 30-minute race. In this example, the maximum sustainable level of exertion for 15 minutes is about 92% of maximum heart rate, compared with about 89% of maximum for 30 minutes. The target heart rates for the endurance/speed and tempo/power workouts are arrayed below the racing levels, with the target rate for the stamina workout anchored at 62% in both cases.

Structuring Tempo Intervals

Some runners are terrible at pacing themselves in a race, partly because they don't structure their intervals properly. In training to build their tempo ability, for instance, they run quarter-mile intervals because that's what they've always run, regardless of whether the resultant tempo is specific to their goal-race.

In other words, the distance and duration of tempo intervals make a difference to the specificity of your pace and heart rate. Since pace-specific tempo training should feel like your current pace for a goal-race, you are looking for an interval distance that enables you to run that pace and finish feeling comfortable. Here's the principle to keep in mind: The shorter the interval the faster you'll tend to run.

If your interval distance is too short, you'll tend to run faster than your racing tempo. And if your interval distance is too long, you'll either run too slowly or too uncomfortably to achieve your tempo training purpose. By experimenting with intervals of various distances (whether 200, 300, 400, 600, or 800 meters, etc.), you'll soon discover an interval that not only feels like your racing tempo but also meets the requisite comfort level. Obviously, finding the right interval distance is a trial and error process. Once you have the right distance, the resultant heart rate will become the target for subsequent workouts. Until then, you are still merely establishing the distance of the interval.

You may have noticed from figures 3.2 and 2.3 that speed and endurance intervals are run at the same target heart rate. This is another example of the principle that interval duration affects race specificity. You can use a relatively long, pace-specific interval for building endurance and a shorter, faster interval for building speed. Both intervals raise exertion to the same target heart rate, but speed intervals raise your heart rate faster because they are specific to a faster surging or kicking pace.

Many runners like to do ladder intervals with a variety of interval distances that build from short to long and down to short again within a workout. This sort of interval structure can bracket your specific race pace with slightly faster and slower running. Since you'll naturally slow down for longer intervals and speed up for shorter intervals, correctly structured ladder interval workouts can combine elements of speed and endurance training while remaining true to the pacing range you could use during a goal-race.

I personally favor tempo workouts that repeat the same interval distance, exclusively. By this method, you could repeat the same interval hundreds of times during a training period of several months, eventually locking into a certain pace so well that you can often predict an interval time to the second. In this case, I think you can appreciate the importance of establishing the right interval distance so you are practicing the right tempo for your goal-race.

Runners who practice their racing tempo extensively will know how to pace themselves when race day arrives. This is a matter of employing the tempo you've often practiced in your training. If that tempo matches your capacity for the race as a whole, you'll run just fast enough in the early going of the race to be comfortable and relaxed. Yet, having maintained the same pace throughout the race, you'll be suitably uncomfortable at the finish.

At this point, you should have a good idea of your exertion for certain workouts, given the race you want to train for and the abilities you want to build in those workouts. You should also have an inkling of how to target your heart rate based on your experience of actually running a new workout. The next step is to actually establish the workout.

Establishing and Monitoring New Workouts

Once you are satisfied that a workout you are planning will achieve your purpose, it's time to run it. Your goal is to establish a set of target heart rate zones. This is a trial and error process that may take several workouts to complete, especially when you have never run a particular workout and you aren't certain about the exact heart rate needed to build an ability.

In this regard, you should have a heart rate monitor so you can track your heart rate during your workouts. You can use the most basic POLAR monitor, or you can get one of the models that enable you to download workout data to a computer. I recommend the more sophisticated models as an investment necessary for effective training. You should have a way of telling exactly how you are structuring your exertion from workout to workout. And using a heart rate monitor with a memory is the best way to track and control the ability-building process.

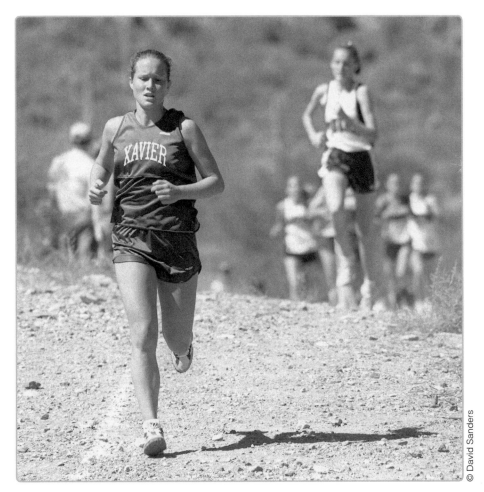

© David Sanders

Endurance is necessary late in the race when it becomes increasingly difficult to maintain your pace against the onset of intensity and fatigue.

Many people find it difficult to cope with the learning curve associated with a new and complex heart rate monitor. If you have read this far, however, you shouldn't have a problem with POLAR's instruction manual! Take your time and learn the monitor in stages. Practice the basics of it and then take the monitor on a run. As you run, you'll probably have difficulty remembering all the functions. Don't be discouraged. You'll learn how to use a monitor eventually, and at that point you'll have control over a powerful training tool.

It's difficult to remember heart rate data unless you have a way to record it during a workout. Ideally, your monitor will have a built-in memory feature that will tell you exactly what your heart rate was from moment to moment during the run. If you have a simpler monitor without a memory feature, you'll need to manually record your heart rate during the workout, stopping just long enough, say, between intervals to record pertinent pace and heart rate data on a laminated form. After the workout you'll have a heart rate record to which you can compare the workout as you planned it.

You should have a clear idea of the exertion level you are aiming for during a workout. Remember, the exertion level is not the same as the target zone. The five abilities are each associated with an exertion level, such as stamina being associated with light exertion or tempo being associated with steady state. Depending on your maximum heart rate, exertion levels can be 15 to 25 beats per minute wide, which is too wide a range for the exact structuring of exertion as we intend it. So, you'll need to narrow your heart rate target the first few times you do a workout.

As you run a workout, you should ask yourself whether your exertion feels too high, too low, or just right. Adjust it so it feels right within the general exertion level. Once you've settled on the right heart rate, the duration of the workout will determine your overall workout effort. Keep playing with the duration of the workout until you have a right-effort workout. Right effort is the combination of effort and energy you've scheduled for yourself. It's also an exertion structure that's consistent with your ability-building purpose, and it's repeatable at an adaptive level.

You may have to run a new workout several times to establish it at a right-effort level. Then notice the exact heart rate structure you've created. It's this structure you should aim to repeat during subsequent workouts. You won't have to change your heart rate targets or the duration of the workout until adaptation has run its course. Meanwhile, the effort of any once-established workout is sufficient for adaptation. All you have to do to build your ability is repeat the workout as established.

Taking the Next Step

At this point, you should have a good idea of your exertion for certain work-outs, given the race you want to train for and the abilities you want to build in those workouts. You should also have an inkling of how to target your heart rate in order to build your racing ability. I'll cover these topics in more detail in chapter 7. Similarly, from chapter 1, you should have an idea of how long your workouts should be. The longer you run at any given heart rate, the harder a workout becomes. Thus, optimal workout duration is just long enough for the amount of energy you have.

In the next chapter, I will ask a related question: how much energy should you have when you go out to do a workout? This question is related to the process of scheduling your workouts during a training week. One way to state the problem is: How do you know when to do a hard workout and when to do an easy one? Understanding how to solve this problem is one of the goals of this book.

CHAPTER 4

Scheduling Workout Effort

The schedules in this chapter don't tell you whether a workout will be long and slow or short and fast. But they will tell you how hard your workouts could be and when you might run them during a normal training week.

This can be a confusing distinction for runners who are used to thinking of a weekly schedule as a prescription to run workouts consisting of pace and mileage. In my system, workouts are fundamentally effort and energy, before pace and mileage. A training schedule refers primarily to workout effort—measured as very easy, easy, moderate, hard, very hard, and all-out.

A training schedule also refers to energy—measured as sluggish, tired, lazy, ready, and eager. Since your energy will change from day to day, a schedule should tell you when to be ready to run your major weekly efforts. In other words, a schedule slots a workout in a certain weekly time slot, and then it tells you when to be recovered from that workout so you can run another workout.

The schedules in this chapter require a certain effort-gauging skill. If you are scheduled to run a *hard* workout, for instance, that's exactly what you must run—not moderate and not very hard. Similarly, if you are scheduled to be *ready* in that hard workout timeslot, then that's exactly how much energy you should have. These skills are acquirable with practice, concentration, and an understanding of basic scheduling concepts.

This chapter includes a number of scheduling alternatives. Some schedules will be more or less appropriate for you, given your individual needs and goals. Please consider the alternatives carefully to choose the one that suits you best.

Scheduling Effort and Recovery

Any time you run, you have an immediate experience of energy–whether it's little energy or abundant energy. The energy is there, whether you are running or not. But you can't experience running energy unless you take a run and feel it.

Metabolic energy cycles determine how much energy you'll have for any run. Sometimes you have ample energy and sometimes you feel like your tank is empty. Since your training affects your energy, the training decisions you make today will affect your energy in the workout or race you do tomorrow. Thus, your races and workouts are all interconnected by metabolic energy cycles.

Using this idea, let's consider a short scheduling problem. Suppose you are planning a new training regimen for your next race, and you've decided to run a hard/ready workout every Sunday morning during the training period (for purposes of this example, you may think of it as a long, slow run). When should you schedule your next hard/ready workout after the Sunday morning run? The simple answer is, when you are ready to run hard again. But the real issue is, *when* will that recovery point occur?

In order to schedule your next workout, you must know how much time you'll need to recover from your previous workout. In general, the harder a workout, the longer its necessary recovery period. Since a typical training schedule can include a range of workout efforts–from very easy to very hard–you'll need to know how much recovery time to schedule after each level of workout effort.

Fortunately, you can predict the time you'll need to recover from a workout, especially if the effort is optimal. Remember from chapter 1: An optimal effort is in harmony with your energy. Taking energy into account, table 4.1 lists the amount of time needed to recover from the five optimal effort/energy combinations.

Let's return to our scheduling problem. According to table 4.1, it takes 48 to 60 hours to recover from a hard/ready workout. If you plan to give yourself the minimum recovery time between hard/ready workouts, you would schedule another hard/ready workout on Tuesday morning–48 hours after the Sunday morning run. Otherwise, you could wait until Tuesday afternoon, which would

TABLE 4.1   Optimal Effort and Recovery Time

Effort/energy combination	Time needed to recover
Very easy/sluggish	< 12 hours
Easy/tired	Approximately 12 hours
Moderate/lazy	24-36 hours
Hard/ready	48-60 hours
Very hard/eager	72-84 hours

be 60 hours after the Sunday run. The time you'll need to recover from a workout depends on its particular combination of effort and energy. By using the information in table 4.1 you can predict your recovery times and schedule your workouts accordingly.

When I recommend scheduling at least 48 to 60 hours between hard workouts, I assume it will take you that long to recover from them. It doesn't matter whether you are an elite athlete or a recreational runner. The recovery periods between your hard workouts should be at least 48 to 60 hours because by definition that's how long it will take you to recover.

Scheduling Recovery Runs

You are recovered from any workout when your energy is sufficient for the effort of the workout you are about to do. Sufficient energy is another way of saying optimal energy. You've got to schedule your recoveries in order to optimize the energy of a workout. In this sense, recovery means returning to a sufficient level of energy.

If your last workout was a hard/ready combination, you are recovered when you are ready-to-run-hard again—not lazy and not eager. Being lazy would give you insufficient energy for a hard workout, while being eager would give you more energy than you need. All you need for a hard workout is to be ready.

Easy Workouts

Suppose you've scheduled two hard workouts 60 hours apart on Sunday morning and Tuesday afternoon. Now it's appropriate to ask whether it's okay to train during the recovery period between these workouts, as well as the other hard workouts on your schedule. Yes, it's okay as long as the interim training doesn't prevent you from being ready-to-run-hard, as scheduled.

In this system, the workouts you do between hard workouts are recovery runs. A recovery run is almost always an easy workout, and easy training is an area of major confusion, as the following questions imply.

> What is the ability-building purpose of easy training?

> How many easy workouts can I schedule between hard workouts?

> Do two easy efforts equal one moderate effort? Or do two 30-minute runs equal a 60-minute run?

> Can easy workouts include cross-training activities, such as swimming, biking, and weightlifting?

First, let's make sure we are on the same page when it comes to the meaning of "easy workout." An easy workout is short *and* slow. That means no more than 30 minutes at mild to light exertion for beginners of little ability, or up to 60 minutes at mild to light exertion for the strongest runners.

An easy workout is not the same as an easy pace. Some runners run a light, "easy" pace for two hours and end up running a moderate-to-hard workout even though they mistakenly call it easy. Similarly, some runners do a short workout on their "easy" days, but they run so fast that the workout also ends up being moderate-to-hard.

This sort of "easy" training breaks the rules of the game. In the hard–easy system, an easy workout is easy–not moderate and certainly not hard. You may be able to do hills and intervals within an easy workout, but the hills and intervals must be light enough that the overall workout is easy. This is not a matter of semantics. Easy means short and slow enough that you recover from the workout in 12 hours.

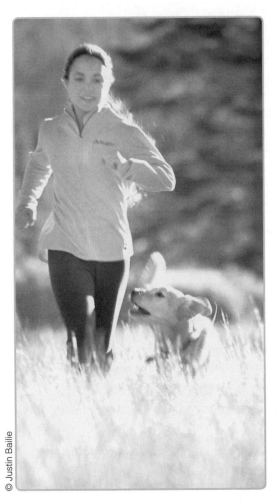

© Justin Bailie

Easy workouts should be relaxed runs—short and slow enough that you recover from them in 12 hours.

No matter whether you are swimming, biking, lifting, or running, it takes discipline to do an easy workout when you have the energy to train harder. No matter how much energy you have, the most important thing is to be faithful to your schedule. If the schedule says to do an easy workout, then that's what you should do because training harder may require you to miss or alter subsequent workouts. Once you begin cutting or missing workouts, the effort stimulus that forms your adaptive base eventually deteriorates.

In the final analysis, your recovery runs should be easy enough to promote regular and adequate recovery from your hard workouts. Regular recovery means you always feel the *same* energy whenever you do a certain hard workout, and adequate recovery means your energy is *sufficient* for the scheduled hard effort.

It's crucial that you have regular and adequate energy every time you do a hard workout. In that way you will know exactly what to expect from those workouts–both in terms of performance and recovery.

Moderate Workouts

Here's another thought problem: Suppose you are scheduled to train at the moderate workout level. How would you know

MY FIRST SCHEDULE

My first experience of scheduling my training occurred in the summer of my sophomore year in college. I was training for a 25K race that summer, and my track coach recommended I do 12-mile runs to prepare, without telling me how to schedule my training.

I had never done distance running before that point of my career. But I had done many interval workouts on successive days so I tried doing 12-mile runs on successive days. I soon discovered that I became increasingly tired with each workout. Then I had to take a day off. After fatiguing myself in this way several times, I came down with a severe cold.

I was smart enough to know that the cold was related to the stress of training, so I decided to change my schedule to avoid the severe fatigue of a third consecutive, hard 12-mile run. I did 12-mile runs on consecutive days, had an off day, followed by another set of two 12-mile runs. Then I completed the week with two off days at the beach.

It wasn't an ideal weekly schedule, but I managed to win a national junior championship 25K race that summer. And I didn't have a recurrence of the cold that had knocked me out of training for a week earlier in the training.

when you've done a moderate workout? It doesn't matter whether you do hills or intervals, or even a certain pace. Rather, it's important that your overall effort is in the moderate range between easy and hard when you end the workout.

But even if you think the effort was moderate, you still won't have it right unless the time you need to recover from it is 24 to 36 hours. If you did the workout feeling lazy and you return to feeling lazy after 24 hours, then it was a moderate workout, especially if you can sustain the same daily workout for weeks or months.

Moderate/lazy workouts are simple to schedule because all you need is one workout that you repeat every day. As uncomplicated as a moderate/lazy schedule is, it can be difficult to gauge the workout effort so your energy returns to lazy every 24 to 36 hours. You could overtrain during a workout and end up feeling tired a day later when you should be lazy. It's always useful, therefore, to have an easy-workout course to fall back on when you feel tired. Generally, you'll know you're tired during the first five minutes of a run, so it could be a simple matter of turning left on your course, instead of right, to shorten the workout and align it with your energy.

Otherwise, with a moderate/lazy regimen, you shouldn't have to worry about scheduling easy runs during extended recovery periods. It's more likely that you'll find small differences in your energy from day to day. Such differences won't necessarily take you out of the lazy range, but they could affect your performances. For instance, when you happen to be on the ready side of lazy for a moderate workout, your pace will reflect this relatively small amount of added energy by being a little faster than usual.

Scheduling Hard Workouts

I am not necessarily advocating hard workouts in this book. Hard training requires an inordinate amount of energy, often more than many responsible adults care to expend. Nonetheless, in the hard–easy system, difficult workouts are the norm.

Hard training is the most effective way to build racing ability at distances between the mile and the marathon. Hard workouts are hard enough to significantly expand your capacity for exertion, while being easy enough to repeat on a reasonably frequent basis.

You can do three hard workouts a week and still recover regularly and adequately, as long as you allow 48 to 60 hours between them, and you don't overtrain. The following schedules address these factors so you can use them to fit your individual circumstances.

Learning Schedule

When you have little or no experience with a particular regimen of hard workouts, it's useful to schedule more than 60 hours to recover from them. I've scheduled as few as one hard workout a week for athletes who are too fragile to do two hard workouts. The rest of the week consists of easy and moderate workouts, with the hard workout being repeated each week on the same day with the same workouts leading up to it.

A single weekly hard workout provides the most basic opportunity to learn how to deal with the stress of hard training. The next step is to develop a schedule with two hard workouts a week. An 84-84-hour hard workout schedule, for instance, gives you exactly half a week (three-and-a-half days or 84 hours) to recover between hard workouts. The 84-84-hour schedule is useful when you are trying to establish new hard workouts and you are uncertain of the amount of running you can do and still recover in 48 to 60 hours.

Scheduling three-and-a-half-day recovery periods isolates each hard workout so you can learn exactly how it is affecting your energy. To find out how a workout is affecting your energy, however, you've got to take a run and feel your energy during a hard workout recovery period. I recommend doing a very-easy-to-easy workout every 12 to 24 hours during an 84-hour recovery period.

The purpose of these recovery runs is to determine exactly when you are sufficiently recovered from your last hard workout. The objective is to gauge the effort of your new hard workouts so you are recovered inside the 84-hour recovery period—ideally at 48 to 60 hours. This should be the time you aim to schedule your recoveries once you've established performance standards for your hard workouts.

A performance standard tells you how much running you can do within a new hard/ready workout. Typically, a standard is couched in terms of a certain number of running minutes at a certain target heart rate. Performance standards take the guesswork out of knowing when you've run a hard workout. In the short-term of a single training period, performance standards tell you almost exactly how much running you can do to maintain the integrity of your schedule.

Advanced Schedule

Once you've established performance standards for several hard workouts, you can integrate them into a tighter, more advanced schedule. The 60-48-60-hour recovery schedule is the most advanced schedule because it gives you minimal recovery time during a week of hard training.

With only 168 hours in a week, and needing a minimum of 48 to 60 hours to recover between hard workouts, you have little leeway to squeeze three hard workouts into one training week. The schedule in figure 4.1 solves this problem by providing 60, 48, and 60 hours between hard workouts.

In this example, the hard workouts are scheduled for Sunday a.m., Tuesday p.m., and Thursday p.m. Though this is a common set of time slots, it's important to realize that you may set up the same 60-48-60-hour schedule in completely different time slots to suit your personal needs and social commitments.

Some people compare the two nights between Sunday and Tuesday with the three nights between Thursday and Sunday and incorrectly assume they have

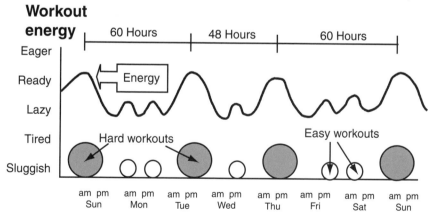

Figure 4.1　This diagram depicts the ebb and flow of energy during the recovery periods between four hard workouts. Energy has a way of rising to the ready level during the last 12 hours of a 48-to-60-hour recovery period. Meanwhile, the easy workouts stimulate the flow of energy during the hard-workout recovery periods, but they aren't hard enough to cause substantial fatigue themselves.

more recovery time during the latter recovery period. While the extra night's sleep may enhance recovery processes, the time between these two sets of hard workouts is still only 60 hours.

The 60-48-60-hour hard workout recovery schedule is effective because it enables you to run three hard workouts in a training week. There are, however, several pitfalls to the schedule. The 48-hour break is hardly enough time to recover from a hard workout, which means you have to be careful running the Tuesday hard workout. A little extra effort on Tuesday could cause you to be lazy instead of ready for the Thursday hard workout, just 48 hours later.

Similarly, it's easy to rationalize a tougher workout on Thursday, knowing you have that extra night's sleep before Sunday. But 60 hours is still only 60 hours. When you are spacing your hard workouts with 48 to 60 hours between them, week after week without a break, they jump up at you in rapid succession—extra sleep not withstanding.

Mixed-Effort Schedule

I used to promote the 60-48-60-hour schedule to runners as a "learning" schedule. They were supposed to learn how their energy fluctuated by feeling how it changed during the easy workouts they were running every 12 hours between hard workouts. Albeit an opportunity for beginners to learn about the ebb and flow of energy, the 60-48-60-hour hard workout schedule is better suited to experienced runners who are able to run three hard workouts a week for months, without breaking down and without making major training mistakes that disrupt their training schedule.

There is little room for error in the 60-48-60-hour hard workout schedule. You must be capable of withstanding the stress of hard training and skilled enough to gauge workout efforts correctly. If you are scheduled to run hard/ready in a certain time slot, for instance, then you must run hard (not moderate or very hard) and you must be ready (not lazy or eager).

As disciplined as you have to be with the 60-48-60-hour schedule, running hard workouts is not your only option. You could run moderate workouts in one or more of the hard workout time slots. Besides providing a lighter training load, a more moderate training regimen can be a stepping stone for building the necessary capacity to train harder later. In this sense, the inclusion of moderate workouts in the hard workout time slots makes the 60-48-60-hour schedule a true learning schedule.

There are other reasons for doing moderate workouts in the hard workout time slots. For one thing, moderate/lazy workouts provide almost as much adaptive value as hard/ready workouts. Moderate workouts can also be a viable alternative when your other time and energy commitments preclude hard training, or when you are out of shape and easing back into running after a long layoff.

Finally, by scheduling moderate workouts as you would hard workouts—with 48 to 60 hours between them—you already have a viable hard workout schedule should you decide to develop your moderate/lazy workouts into hard/ready workouts.

Morning or Evening Schedule

Some people don't like the 60-48-60-hour schedule because it places at least one hard workout in the morning and the evening each week. As an alternative, you could run all of your hard workouts in the morning or evening to suit your personal needs.

I recommend a 48-48-72-hour schedule to meet the goal of running three hard workouts per week in the morning or evening only. The disadvantage of this schedule is having minimal, 48-hour recovery periods after two consecutive hard workouts each week. Since it's difficult to sustain a schedule that permits only 48 hours between hard workouts, this schedule affords a 72-hour recovery period once a week so you can recover more thoroughly before beginning the same schedule the following week.

Adjusting to an Energy Shortfall

As I indicated in the previous section, establishing performance standards is part of setting up a new workout. A performance standard can be as simple as running a certain number of miles at a certain heart rate.

A target heart rate is not an end in itself. Target heart rates are meant to guide you in structuring workouts to achieve an ability-building purpose. But they don't necessarily point at *right* exertion. Right exertion is optimal exertion, which depends on how your running energy changes during a workout.

Depending on how much energy you have (none, little, some, ample, or abundant), right exertion might feel satisfying, enjoyable, or exhilarating. The harder you run beyond right exertion, the more dissonance you experience, which increases the risk of getting injured or becoming rapidly fatigued. An effective way to measure dissonance is to consider your attitude about the effort you are exerting.

Effort Attitude Scale

Exhilarated: Feeling of supreme well-being, including mild euphoria.

Enjoyed: Pleasant, pleasurable, delightful, or fun.

Satisfied: Okay; neither positive nor negative.

Burdened: Duty-bound to perform, unpleasant.

Oppressed: Detestable drudgery.

It's never okay to feel burdened or oppressed by a workout. Burdensome running always has negative repercussions that can ultimately take you completely out of the competitive game. Of course, it's okay occasionally during a compelling, competitive racing event to feel burdened by your effort, as long as you also realize that you could pay certain prices as a result. But being constantly burdened by your training is downright destructive to adaptive processes.

So, which is more effective: to run a target heart rate at a burdensome level or to run a slower, more satisfying pace in harmony with your energy? Your answer to this question will determine the amount of adaptive value you derive from your training. Let's consider a short case study to illustrate my point.

This study focuses on Dana, a 30-year-old woman athlete in one of my programs, and the hard/ready, 1,200-meter interval workout she was doing under my supervision. The purpose of Dana's workout was to build a base of quick and relaxed tempo running that approached her audible breathing threshold. By repeating the workout from week to week, she intended to consolidate her ability at that steady-state level before developing a new, pace-specific workout for the 10K goal-race she aimed to do in five months.

I worked with Dana for several weeks while she established the workout. Once established, she had the following performance standards to aim at during the rest of her 10-week training period. First, she aimed to run the tempo intervals within a target zone of 155 to 159 beats per minute. Second, she aimed to do eight 1,200-meter intervals by the time noticeable fatigue set in. Third, every time she was scheduled to do the workout, she aimed to be ready-to-run-hard.

In an ideal world, Dana could have counted on being ready-to-run-hard every time she was scheduled to run this workout. From her experience of establishing the workout, she knew that when she had ample energy early in the workout she could run eight 1,200-meter intervals, with noticeable fatigue setting in on the last interval, providing she also stayed within her target zone. Running above that zone caused premature fatigue, which would force her to end the workout before she had run her quota of eight intervals.

When Dana had abundant energy—the level above ample—she had to hold herself back to stay within her target zone. She knew that being eager would enable her to run more intervals at a faster pace. Since the quality of her performance would determine her workout effort, a tremendous performance would lead to an extended recovery period. Thus, having too much energy was one pitfall she was concerned about before her major workouts.

Occasionally, Dana would also have to deal with less energy than she needed. This was true of the 1,200-meter interval workout she ran on the fifth week of her training period. Though she was ready for the workout, she was on the low side of ready—closer to lazy than eager. As a result, she struggled through the first 10 minutes of the workout, warming up slowly and feeling only some energy instead of the usual ample energy at the end of 12 minutes.

As she started her first interval, she realized immediately that she would have a difficult time getting her heart rate into the target zone. She could press the pace to 155 BPM, but she knew intuitively her exertion would be harsh, jarring, and discordant. Thus, she had a decision to make: She could press the pace to her usual target heart rate or she could stay relaxed at a lower heart rate and a slower pace.

As an intermediate athlete with good natural talent, Dana was very pace conscious. Other runners had told her that sometimes she would have to push the pace in a race when her energy wasn't good. From their perspective, she had to get used to pushing through similar rough spots in her training; otherwise, she couldn't do it in her races. Fortunately, she had my perspective for comparison. I believe training and racing are the same when it comes to exerting harmonious efforts. In a race, I always wait for my energy to develop before pushing the pace, even when it means falling behind competitively. Notwithstanding having to gut it out at the end of close races, there are always prices to pay for running races dissonantly.

Whether we are willing to pay those prices depends on our mental toughness and our will to win in the defining moment of a race. We don't have to abuse ourselves in training to know how to abuse ourselves competitively. Since Dana wasn't into abusive training, she focused on running quick and relaxed, albeit at a slower tempo. By the fourth interval, she had warmed up well enough that she was feeling ample energy and running in her target zone. Unfortunately, her energy was never as good as it would have been at the ready level. As a result, she ran into early fatigue during the seventh interval. At that point, her pace slowed slightly and she had trouble keeping her heart rate from rising above the target zone—a sign of noticeable fatigue.

Now, she had another decision to make. The eighth interval was right there to be run, or shunned. Her friends would have advised completing the workout to prepare for those inevitable competitive moments when mental toughness would determine who won or lost a tight race. My words rang truer: to hurt her running

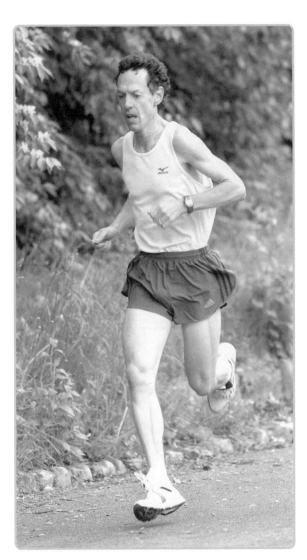

Even if you start a race with abundant energy, fatigue eventually sets in and requires you to approach the limit of your capacity for exertion.

spirit with disagreeable training was to hurt it for her goal-race. Not wanting to overtrain, Dana decided to end the workout feeling satisfied, rather than pushing to finish the eighth interval feeling burdened.

What's the lesson to be learned here? Whether you actually hit a target heart rate should depend on whether your energy allows it in the moment. Thus, we can visualize the possibility of a *curved* target zone that fits the movement of one's energy as it changes during a workout (see figure 4.2).

Dana knew from experience that a lack of energy increases resistance to the effort of a run, and that fighting this resistance to maintain her pace and heart rate would counteract her adaptive purpose. Thus, she slowed down in the early going of the workout to accommodate her less-than-adequate energy, and she increased her heart rate only as her energy developed to the ample level. When her pace slowed on the seventh interval, she realized that she was getting fatigued. Since she wanted to keep her overall effort at the optimal, hard workout level, she ended the workout before the eighth interval.

This low-energy syndrome is common to all sorts of workouts, not only interval workouts. You should be on guard during all your workouts, therefore, for signs of fatigue so you can adjust your performance to accommodate your energy. It's always better in low-energy circumstances to do less than more.

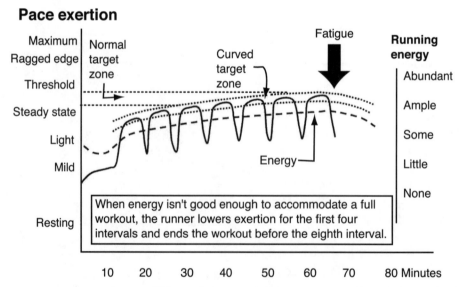

Figure 4.2 During the first 30 minutes of the workout, the runner's energy rose from *some* to *ample*. As her energy improved to its usual *ample* level, her target zone rose to its usual level, too. During the seventh interval, however, her pace slowed and she had trouble keeping her heart rate in the target zone. Taking this as a sign of notice-able fatigue, she ended the workout before the eighth interval.

Assessing Your Current Schedule

Take some time now to think about your current workout schedule. You might think that you don't have a regular schedule, because you don't have a regular training routine. Nonetheless, for your assessment purposes, please answer the following questions according to a distribution of workouts from one of your recent training weeks, one that approximates the overall amount of effort you typically exert.

> **Assessing Your Current Weekly Schedule.** The main reason for doing this exercise is to develop an estimate of your current capacity for weekly training effort. You will use this estimate in chapters 7 and 8 should you decide to take on a new set of workouts, along with a new weekly schedule and a new training program. Table 4.2 gives you a way to plot your current training schedule in terms of when and how hard you run during a training week. This schedule should plot the overall effort of each workout, not the specific activities you do such as hills or intervals.

In filling out table 4.2, please use the following terms and abbreviations for each workout you do: very easy (VE), easy (E), moderate (M), hard (H), very hard (VH), or all-out (AO). If these terms are unfamiliar to you, you can review the pertinent section of chapter 1 and the workout effort scale on page 8.

Place your workouts in the appropriate time slots. If you don't have a regular schedule, see about approximating when and how hard you run during a typical week. Also, please circle the efforts you consider to be your major weekly workouts.

TABLE 4.2 Current Weekly Training Schedule

	Sun	Mon	Tue	Wed	Thu	Fri	Sat
a.m.							
Noon							
p.m.							

> **Assessing Your Current Capacity for Weekly Training.** Figure 4.3 will assist you in analyzing your weekly schedule to determine your capacity for exertion. Notice that your answer to each question falls on a scale that measures your capacity from high to low. By answering all seven questions you should get a picture of your capacity for weekly training effort, which you can use in later chapters to set up an effective training program.

Figure 4.3

Assessing Your Capacity
for Weekly Training

1. *Number of Workouts.* How many running workouts are you currently doing on a regular weekly basis?

Workouts	Capacity
_____ 1-4	Low
_____ 5-10	Medium
_____ 10-14	High

2. *Double Workouts.* How many times a week do you run twice a day?

Doubles	Capacity
_____ 0	Low
_____ 1-4	Medium
_____ 5-7	High

3. *Days Off.* How many days a week do you take off from running?

Days Off	Capacity
_____ 0-1	High
_____ 2	Medium
_____ 3-4	Low

4. *Weekly Mileage.* During the past six months, what was your average *weekly* mileage (running or jogging consistently)?

Mileage	Capacity
_____ 0-19	Low
_____ 20-49	Medium
_____ 50-70+	High

5. *Three Hardest Optimal Workouts.* Please return to the five-question process you completed at the end of chapter 1. Repeat that process for the next two hardest workouts on your current weekly schedule. This will give you a clear idea of the effort of the three hardest workouts you do on a weekly basis.

   Assuming your three hardest workouts are optimal effort/energy combinations (i.e., you aren't running too hard or too easily in relation to your energy), this is another way to estimate your capacity for exertion (see table 4.3).

From *5K and 10K Training* by Brian Clarke, 2006, Champaign, IL: Human Kinetics.

TABLE 4.3 Capacity Based on Three Hardest Weekly Workouts

	THREE HARDEST WORKOUTS		
	#1	#2	#3
LOW	Easy	Easy	Easy
	Easy	Easy	Moderate
	Easy	Moderate	Moderate
MEDIUM	Moderate	Moderate	Moderate
	Easy	Easy	Hard
	Easy	Moderate	Hard
HIGH	Moderate	Moderate	Hard
	Easy	Hard	Hard
	Moderate	Hard	Hard
	Hard	Hard	Hard

6. *Average Workout Effort (All Weekly Workouts).* What's the average workout effort for all the workouts on your schedule? Here's how to calculate average effort if, for example, you are doing four moderate workouts and two hard workouts a week:

Multiply the number of workouts in each effort category by its effort level (i.e., very easy = 1, easy = 2, moderate = 3, hard = 4, and very hard = 5). Thus, if you run 4 moderate workouts and 2 hard workouts, the calculations are: $4 \times 3 = 12$, and $2 \times 4 = 8$.

Then add all workout effort points and divide by the total number of workouts you do in a week. Again, if you run 4 moderate workouts and 2 hard workouts, your efforts add up to $12 + 8 = 20$. Thus, your average effort level is 20 divided by 6 = 3.33, meaning your average workout effort is between moderate and hard.

Average Effort	Capacity
2.4 or less	Low
2.5 to 3.4	Medium
3.5 or more	High

(continued)

From *5K and 10K Training* by Brian Clarke, 2006, Champaign, IL: Human Kinetics.

Figure 4.3 *(continued)*

7. *Workout Structure (Your Hardest Weekly Workout).* Next, let's consider the exertion structure of the hardest workout you currently do on a regular, weekly basis. How long is that workout in minutes? Please circle that number in the duration column of table 4.4. Note: workout duration does not include a 10-minute warm-up and a 5-minute cool-down.

TABLE 4.4 Your Hardest Weekly Workout

Workout duration (minutes)	High (H), Medium (M), and Low (L) capacity at average level of exertion (between warm-up and cool-down)					
10	Mild (L)	Light (L)	Steady (L)	Threshold (M)	Ragged (M)	Max (H)
20	Mild (L)	Light (L)	Steady (L)	Threshold (M)	Ragged (H)	Max (H)
30	Mild (L)	Light (L)	Steady (M)	Threshold (M)	Ragged (H)	
40	Mild (L)	Light (L)	Steady (M)	Threshold (H)	Ragged (H)	
50	Mild (L)	Light (L)	Steady (M)	Threshold (H)	Ragged (H)	
60	Mild (L)	Light (M)	Steady (M)	Threshold (H)	Ragged (H)	
70	Mild (L)	Light (M)	Steady (H)	Threshold (H)	Ragged (H)	
80	Mild (M)	Light (M)	Steady (H)	Threshold (H)	Ragged (H)	
90	Mild (M)	Light (M)	Steady (H)	Threshold (H)		
100	Mild (M)	Light (H)	Steady (H)			
110	Mild (M)	Light (H)	Steady (H)			
120	Mild (M)	Light (H)	Steady (H)			
120-180	Mild (M)	Light (H)				

From *5K and 10K Training* by Brian Clarke, 2006, Champaign, IL: Human Kinetics.

Estimating Your Hardest
Current Workout Structure

Please also circle the average level of exertion for the workout, whether mild, light, steady state, or threshold. Note: Average level of exertion for the workout does not include a 10-minute warm-up and 5-minute cool-down. If you are running intervals, however, it does include the exertion of your tempo interval averaged with the exertion of your rest interval.

In other words, if your average heart rate from the first interval to the last interval, including rest breaks, is 74 percent of maximum, then your average for the workout is steady state, which encompasses the heart rate range between 70 and 79 percent of maximum (see the components of exertion scale on page 2).

Next, on table 4.4, notice your estimated capacity, whether low (L), medium (M), or high (H), based on the duration and exertion level of your hardest current workout.

At this point, you have seven different factors for estimating your capacity for exertion. None of these factors by itself will give you a complete picture of your capacity. But considered together they should give you a solid basis for estimating your capacity. Using your scores for the seven factors in this section, please circle your scores for each factor listed below.

	Capacity		
Number of workouts	Low	Medium	High
Double workouts	Low	Medium	High
Off-days	Low	Medium	High
Weekly mileage	Low	Medium	High
Three hardest optimal workouts	Low	Medium	High
Average workout effort	Low	Medium	High
Workout structure (hardest workout)	Low	Medium	High

For your programmatic purposes in later chapters, your capacity for exertion is the score you've given yourself most often. Thus, for example, in the unlikely event that you had two lows, two highs, and three mediums, then you have a medium capacity.

From *5K and 10K Training* by Brian Clarke, 2006, Champaign, IL: Human Kinetics.

Taking the Next Step

The schedules suggested in this chapter provide a framework within which your training could occur. If you don't understand how to work within that framework, your training could do more harm than good. Thus, even before you begin to train, you must understand the scheduling problem. The scheduling problem can be summed up with two questions: *When* should I train? And how *hard* should I train? Whether you were aware of it or not, you've answered these questions every time you've ever done a workout. However, providing an answer is not the same as providing a viable solution. How many times, for instance, have you hurt yourself by running your workouts out of convenience or impulse?

Understanding how to schedule your workouts is one of the basic problems of the training process. And viable solutions are the necessary prerequisite for effective training. This chapter has provided you with the concepts necessary to schedule your workouts within a week of training. In the next chapter, I will step back and consider some ideas that affect your training on a month-to-month basis.

CHAPTER 5

Balancing Effort and Fatigue

Why do so many runners become sick, injured, or exhausted just before a major racing event? The quick and easy answer is that overtraining has negative consequences, including injury, illness, and exhaustion. The longer, more difficult answer requires a more comprehensive understanding of the training process.

Training is what we do when we repeat a workout regimen. Our workouts are adaptive stimuli that affect our capacity for exertion. During a training period leading up to a goal-race, our capacity alternately contracts and expands in response to metabolic forces beyond our direct control. This is why endurance training is so beguiling; we can't simply train and expect adaptation to occur automatically.

Adaptive training is the process of getting our workouts right, and right effort is always a moving target. In the short term of weekly training, right effort depends on adjusting your effort to your energy as it fluctuates from day to day. In the long term of a 12-week training period, it depends on adjusting your effort according to the major phases of the training cycle.

The Three Phases of Training

In the 1950s, Hans Selye established the tenets of a new theory of adaptation in his book *The Stress of Life*. According to Selye, all living organisms react in three phases to any of life's stressors. Selye termed the phases shock, adaptation, and exhaustion (see figure 5.1). Together, these ideas explain what happens to any endurance athlete in pursuit of improved racing performance.

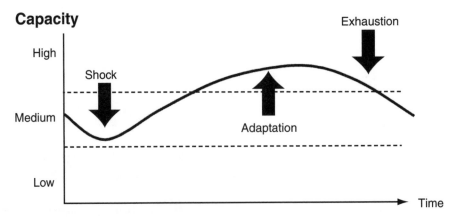

Figure 5.1 Hans Selye showed that any living organism goes through three phases in response to the stress of a new and constant life event. The phases are shock, adaptation, and exhaustion, which Selye termed the General Adaptation Syndrome. According to Selye, adaptation is not immediate or inevitable. Rather, the initial stress of a life event could shock the organism into reduced capacity or even death. Similarly, adaptation once begun was not interminable. Thus, according to Selye, all organisms eventually run out of adaptive energy and become exhausted.

Selye's theory predicts that a runner's performance capacity will shrink in response to a new workout regimen. As a result of shock, workouts we ordinarily consider within our capacity become too difficult as our body reacts to the stress of novel training effort. This shock phase of training has to be accounted for whenever we begin a new training regimen.

Unless we exert the right effort in response to the shock of novel training, we can experience myriad stress symptoms, including colds and injuries, irritability, insomnia, lack of appetite, diarrhea, and for females, disruption of the menstrual cycle. The time it takes to recover from these afflictions delays the process of establishing a new workout.

Establishing a New Workout

The process of establishing a new workout is one of the most difficult aspects of the training process. How hard should the workout be to minimize the inevitable shock of novel effort? Most authorities advise us to start off slow and easy. But exactly what is slow and easy in this context? What rules, standards, or concepts apply? The complexities are overwhelming.

Ultimately, surviving the shock of novel effort is a matter of exerting the easiest effort consistent with your ability-building purpose. Any workout will be designed to build one of five abilities: stamina, power, tempo, speed, and endurance. There is a certain amount of planning required to develop the exertion structure of a new workout. And you should have that structure in mind when you first run the workout so you can conform to its ability-building purpose.

You should also know how the overall effort of the workout will fit within your current capacity for exertion so you can avoid throwing yourself severely into shock. Consider, for example, the case of John, a 30-year-old recreational runner who came to me for advice after a disastrous 10K race. In some ways, he thought his preparation had been ideal, but the race went poorly because he was suffering from the effects of a bad cold he had contracted the week before the race.

John had wanted to establish a new tempo workout at the beginning of the 13-week training period leading up to his 10K. He was concerned about it because had never trained at his planned tempo heart rate, and he had never trained at the hard workout level. The hardest workouts he was used to running were light-to-steady-state, moderate workouts. The prospect of running the new tempo workout was troublesome to him because he suspected it would throw him into shock.

Figure 5.2 illustrates John's problem. The essence of the problem was the difference between his current capacity and the capacity he needed to run the new workout. Since the new workout was projected to be 60 minutes long, it would be at least as hard as his current moderate workout, which was also 60 minutes. Clearly the higher exertion level of the intervals would make the new workout harder than the old, but until he had run the workout, he wouldn't know exactly how much additional stress it might generate.

In thinking about the new workout ahead of time, John had decided to fix the duration of his tempo intervals at about five minutes. Five minutes would give him enough time to raise his heart rate gradually during each interval, and it

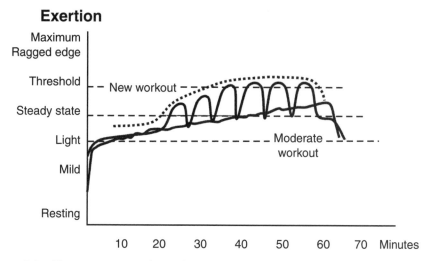

Figure 5.2 There are two workouts juxtaposed in this graph: an established 60-minute, light-to-steady moderate workout (bottom curve), and a new workout (top curve), with six 5-minute tempo intervals at the runner's lowest audible breathing level. If both workouts are the same duration, the new workout must be harder because its volume—the area under the dotted curve—is greater than the volume for the moderate workout.

would also give him enough time to practice sustaining his specific racing tempo before he gave himself a 90-second rest. Since the duration of the intervals was set at five minutes, the major factor affecting the overall workout effort would be the number of intervals completed during the workout. In John's mind, the main issue was whether to run four, five, or six intervals to start.

Knowing he had little experience with the workout, he decided to run four intervals the first time he did the workout. He also decided to run the intervals at a somewhat lower heart rate than the one he planned to run once he'd established the workout. On that basis, the first workout took 45 minutes, and John rated it as a little harder than the moderate run he was used to doing. In my opinion, John had done the right thing. By lowering his exertion and limiting the number of intervals, he kept the overall effort of the new interval workout within a manageable range. And although he experienced some pain and stiffness after the workout, he didn't need to take time off.

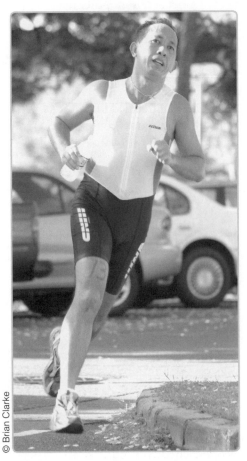

© Brian Clarke

Ease into new workouts, giving your body time to adjust to the shock of novel training effort.

The next week, John added one five-minute interval to the workout, and he increased his tempo heart rate by an average of one beat per minute. Again, he was able, with minimal soreness, to recover in time for his next workout. By this step-by-step method, he gradually increased the effort of the workout, giving himself time to establish it at the hard/ready level by the fourth week.

Balancing Right Effort and Right Fatigue

Some experienced runners wouldn't have had the patience to start as conservatively as John did with his new tempo workout. Unfortunately, the longer it has been since they ran a workout, the harder it is to estimate their right starting effort. They think they know what's right, but their ambition entices them to bite off more than they can chew.

John, by contrast, realized that his hardest current workout wasn't as hard as his new workout was projected to be. He was used to running moderate workouts, but the new workout would require a larger capacity. Figure 5.2 is a way of visualizing the sort of capacity he needed for the new workout. Since his capacity was right for the moderate workouts he was doing, he reasoned, doing a hard

THE GENERAL ADAPTATION SYNDROME

I like to introduce the topic of adaptation by telling my students about a white rat experiment. Scientists have long used white rats to understand human behavior and physiology. The scientists in this imaginary experiment had a large vat of ice cold water in their laboratory. At the beginning of the experiment they placed 100 rats in the water and allow them to swim around for several hours. At the end of that time they took the rats out, dried them off, and placed them in their cages for the rest of the day.

The next day the scientists put the rats in the cold water again, repeating the process every day for a week. At the end of the week, they counted 30 rats that had died from intermittent exposure to the cold water. Each of these rats was autopsied and discovered to have an excess of hormone "A" in their blood. When the scientists sampled the blood of the 70 living rats, they discovered their blood also had an excess of hormone "A."

During the following week, only 10 rats died, and all of them had excessive amounts of hormone "A" in their blood. The other 60 rats, however, were discovered to have little hormone "A" at this juncture. Instead, their blood was replete with hormone "B." At the end of the second week, seeing the decreased incidence of death and the appearance of hormone "B," the scientists wondered whether the remaining rats might be able to survive their daily cold water swim. But during the third week something happened they didn't anticipate: All the remaining rats died, and they all had a surfeit of hormone "A" in their blood.

At this point, the scientists had the task of explaining what had happened—not only during the final week but for the experiment as a whole. This problem is similar to the one that a pioneering theoretical scientist, Hans Selye, faced in the early 1950s when he was conducting similar experiments to understand what he termed the *General Adaptation Syndrome*. You can find more information about similar experiments in Selye's book *The Stress of Life*.

workout initially would probably be more than he could handle when it came to his available training energy.

In establishing the new workout, he decided to adjust his initial effort to the amount of energy he knew he'd have. Getting the energy of a new workout right is tied up with getting fatigue right. Fatigue is a necessary aspect of the training process. You can't improve without encountering fatigue, both during your workouts and between them. With a new workout, it's difficult to anticipate the exact point when you'll become appropriately fatigued. Once you've actually run the workout, however, your experience will tell you whether you ended the workout at the right level of fatigue.

Because you have limited time to train before a goal-race, it is wise to ease progressively into your new workouts the first several times you do them. This may sound paradoxical but remember, it's always better initially to run the least effort compatible with the ability-building purpose of a new workout, so you can recover for your next workout without crashing. If you are establishing a stamina workout, for example, stay within your light exertion range but keep to the lower end of it. If you are aiming for a hard workout, keep to the moderate side of hard by abbreviating the workout while you are establishing it.

It's important to realize that adaptation doesn't begin until you've established a new workout and you've weathered the shock of doing something new. At that point, an optimal effort can expand your performance capacity without causing injury, illness, or premature exhaustion. Until then you are only establishing the workout.

Preventing Overtraining

Assuming you've established a new workout, you should begin to show some positive changes in your capacity. By repeating the workout as established, ideally you'll reach peak ability on race day. In the real world, however, the ideal is often just beyond our reach, which is why it's so tempting to overreach.

Consider John's experience of doing his new tempo workout during the second half of the 13-week training period leading up to his 10K race. By week four, the workout consisted of six 1,200-meter tempo intervals, each lasting about five minutes. By week six his tempo pace had dropped to 6:30 per mile. Not only had his pace improved from workout to workout, but he also felt increasingly proficient.

Proficiency is a sense of one's ability to do a workout as measured on the following scale: *unable, ineffective, passably able, effective, fully able*. Proficiency includes the feeling of strength and confidence that comes with successfully repeating a workout as scheduled. In the early weeks of John's 13-week training period, he'd been only passably able to do the tempo workout. Then, for a couple of weeks, he knew he could do it effectively. By the seventh week, there was no doubt in his mind that he was fully able do the workout.

During our subsequent coaching discussion, John's week-seven experience stood out in his mind because he was eager to do that workout. Feeling eager, he pushed the pace under 6:30 per mile—flying along as he had never flown before, even in his fastest 10Ks. Later, he thought he may have pushed too hard, because he was forced to take a day off to recover from a sore Achilles tendon. He was also unusually tired from the workout, and his lack of energy negatively affected his performances during his workouts for about a week.

John also thought he had peaked too soon. In the eighth week he was ready to do the workout, but he didn't run as fast as he had the week before. Anxious about his ability, he pressed to maintain a sub-6:30 pace. During the next several weeks, he continued to add exertion in order to maintain his pace in response to what he perceived to be dwindling energy. He still felt ready to run a hard workout, but he didn't have enough energy to sustain his week-seven pace.

His proficiency seemed to have deteriorated. He didn't feel as strong or confident as he had been at his peak in week seven. In week 11, after an extended 72-hour recovery period, he ran a very hard/ready workout, maintaining the sub-6:30 pace he had held with the hard/eager workout four weeks earlier (see figure 5.3).

At that point, it finally dawned on John that something was wrong. The same rapid, pressing, sub-6:30 pace that felt so exhilarating only four weeks earlier was now a burden to him. Meanwhile, his heart rate had risen an average of five beats per minute and his legs simply didn't have the snap they had in week seven. With only two weeks remaining before his goal-race, John had a decision to make. How could he correct the difficulty he had created for himself?

John decided it was time to follow the two-week taper plan he had scheduled for himself at the start of the training period. Three days later, he began feeling the symptoms of a mild cold. Thinking he should get in one more tempo workout before cutting back to easy workouts, he ran the workout 10 days before the race. Several days later, John developed a severe cough, which markedly diminished his prospects for a good race experience.

One of the most difficult things to accept about life is the inevitability of exhaustion. No endurance athlete can expect to maintain a high level of adaptation indefinitely. John made a mistake in week eight by pressing to maintain a

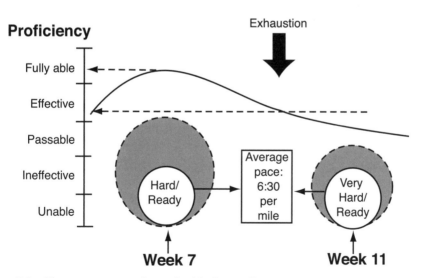

Figure 5.3 There are two workouts in this figure. Both workouts consist of an outer circle that represents capacity and an inner circle that represents effort. Both were run at the same average pace of 6:30 per mile. The workout in week 11 is harder than the one in week 7 because exhaustion has reduced capacity from *fully able* to *barely effective*.

HAVING A BASE

One of my best friends, Akabill Molmen, continued to improve all of his times through his 40s and 50s on the strength of his enthusiasm for progressively longer training runs. In the early 1980s, I was a significantly faster runner than Akabill. During the next 20 years, however, I spent a lot of time recovering from injuries, while Akabill became one of Hawaii's foremost ultramarathoners.

At his best in the early 2000s, Akabill regularly ran 40- to 60-mile trail runs on the weekend with a "short" mid-week 20-mile road and trail run through some of the hilliest rainforest in the Hawaiian Islands. In the late 1990s, we raced the Kilauea Volcano Wilderness Marathon, and Akabill beat me by 45 minutes. A year later, while training for the Angeles Crest 100-miler,

he ran the Volcano Marathon, the 10-mile Crater Rim Run, and the 5-mile Caldera Run consecutively, and he still beat me in the marathon.

Few people have Akabill's enthusiasm, persistence, and toughness, which is why few people reach their running potential. Interestingly, by building a huge base of stamina, Akabill also expanded his capacity for steady-state running. He never did intervals or speed work, yet he could race effectively at a higher level of exertion than the one at which he built his base. So don't feel you always have to train specifically.

Your capacity for long, slow running readily converts to faster running whenever you choose to run at a quicker pace. And that higher-level capacity for exertion will be greater than it would have been without the benefit of prior base building.

---

sub-6:30 pace. Exhaustion was setting in then, but he was either unwilling or unable to see it coming. During subsequent workouts, he continued to push against exhaustion in a vain attempt to maintain his pace performance.

There is absolutely no way we can improve performance capacity by pushing against exhaustion. The harder we push with workout effort, the harder exhaustion pushes back at us. So what could John have done in week eight when he first noticed that his energy wasn't going to allow him to sustain his pace with the same ease of the previous week? Would it have helped to run a slower pace while maintaining the same heart rate as before? Of course, this would have been a better choice than increasing his heart rate to maintain peak performance.

By backing off on effort in the eighth week, John might have staved off the full effect of exhaustion through the rest of the training period. There's a tendency for capacity to plateau after hitting a peak, as long as you maintain an established level of effort. The new performance level won't be as high as the recent peak, but it's usually much higher than the level you started with at the beginning of the training period. In John's case, certainly his proficiency would have been greater a week before his goal-race than the ineffective level he was experiencing with the bad cold.

It's also interesting to consider whether John might have done something to avoid the cold. With exhaustion clearly at an advanced stage two weeks before his goal-race, he didn't have time for a gradual taper. He should have resisted the urge to do one more tempo workout, while doing nothing more than easy workouts until race day.

Repeating Workouts to Increase Capacity

I mentioned that John made a mistake by pressing to maintain his pace in the eighth week of his training period. This was an indication of a misplaced focus. Rather than focusing on his pace, he should have focused on his exertion. Remember, exertion is the adaptive stimulus, not pace.

The most objective form that exertion takes is a target heart rate. How do you know when you've targeted the *right* heart rate? The right heart rate depends on the way your exertion feels in relation to your energy. In fact, unless you have a lot of recent experience with the same workout, setting a target heart rate is a matter of running the workout until it feels right, then noticing the heart rate that made it feel right.

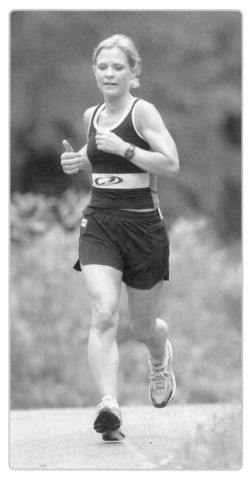

Exhaustion is inevitable in the training context. Thus, the goal of training is to avoid severe exhaustion by staying well within your capacity for exertion.

You are feeling for specific levels of exertion, energy, and fatigue. And you're attempting to match these feelings with an idea of the ability you want to build. You haven't established the workout until everything feels right, and feeling right is not the same as feeling good. There's no question that flying along when you have abundant energy feels good. But you aren't supposed to have abundant energy when you are only allowing yourself ample energy for your major workouts. Moreover, it's a pitfall to believe that you can run harder than your target heart rate because you feel better than usual.

The discipline of training requires you to run the boring right effort, often at the expense of the more exhilarating feel-good effort. The mantra to repeat is this: *I save my energy for the races*. We want our races to be exhilarating because that's one of the best aspects of the game. By comparison, training is often only satisfying, and only sometimes enjoyable. Feeling exhilarated by a workout usually means that you've taken too much rest before the run and, as a result, you feel eager to race. So you race along because it feels good. But, afterwards, while you suffer through a minor injury or an extended recovery period, you wonder why you wasted all that energy on a workout.

It's better to run consistently. Consistency is like baking a cake. The baking process requires that you mix the dry and liquid ingredients correctly, so the cake is neither too dry nor too moist. Similarly, with training you have to mix your effort and your energy consistently to stimulate and prolong adaptation.

Too little effort and you won't adapt; too much effort and you'll crash, either from shock or exhaustion. It's crucial, therefore, that you maintain the consistency of an adaptive effort by repeating your workouts as established.

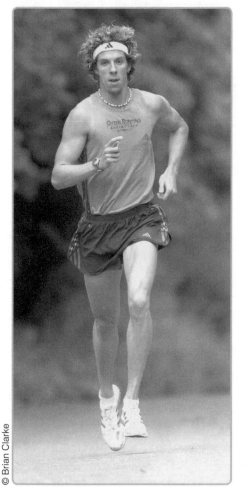

Every workout carries with it the risk of injury. Harmonious effort is an optimal balance of potential adaptive gains and the unavoidable risk of injury.

© Brian Clarke

The Three Training Objectives

There are three objectives to every training period: to minimize shock, maximize adaptation, and avoid severe exhaustion. If you are like me in your desire to master endurance training, you must ask yourself a pertinent question: What aspects of the training process can you manipulate to achieve these objectives?

Every time you run a workout, you deal with effort and energy. But unless you are consciously coordinating your efforts with your energy, improved performance happens as much by accident as by design. Some competitive runners are accustomed to thinking in terms of performance, while overlooking their dynamic capacity for exertion. Ultimately, we must make our capacity the main focus of our training. This mental shift requires a radically different training perspective.

Ordinarily, pace and mileage are the standards by which we judge our training between races. Yet, there are metabolic repercussions whenever our pace and mileage are inappropriate for the amount of energy we have. Adaptation is our main objective, and we are adapting as long as our performance capacity improves without injury, illness, or exhaustion.

Taking the Next Step

We are all interested in how we can make our capacity grow from month to month so we can perform better in our races. This chapter has dealt with ideas related to the broad view of training on a month-to-month basis. The forces that determine this long term improvement are shock, adaptation and exhaustion. These are metabolic forces that are not directly within our purview. As a result, we may be training, but our effort is not necessarily having the right results because our training is being governed by a metabolic force that's contracting our capacity, rather than expanding it. This is the context within which you must understand the next several chapters on the process of programmatic training. How can we string a long series of workouts together to increase our performance capacity for a goal-race?

CHAPTER 6

Programming Your Training

For some time now, periodic training has been a popular subject in the running literature. Most authors view the topic from the perspective of workout regimens, and how they change on a periodic basis. This book is different in one significant way: It juxtaposes training periods with training cycles.

If a training period is the timeframe within which a workout regimen will be repeated, a training cycle is the physical effect of repeating that regimen. Every training cycle has the potential for shock, adaptation, and exhaustion. We must learn to coordinate our workout efforts with these metabolic forces to achieve our ability-building purposes. This is the essence of the programmatic game, and the new frontier on the way to effective training.

Playing a winning programmatic game means that each workout regimen we establish leads eventually to peak performance in a goal-race. But how can we be sure that our workouts will affect our metabolism according to our intended, periodic timeframe? Without apparent rhyme or reason our capacity sometimes shrinks, leaving us injured or exhausted at the most inopportune moments. We have no guarantee that any workout will increase our performance capacity, because doing workouts is not the same as making adaptive progress with them.

Building a Training Base

It's interesting how different coaches have completely opposite rationales for periodic training. Some begin with short, fast training and build duration; others use the opposite approach. I've been most successful with the Lydiard approach of building stamina first and working for speed later. I like the logic of that approach. I like its symmetry and, ultimately, I like its results.

Unfortunately, Lydiard's system has become associated with 100-mile training weeks. The goal of building to 100 miles a week, not to mention starting at that level, is unrealistic for most recreational athletes. Lydiard, we must remember, worked mostly with young, elite athletes. Nonetheless, somewhere between 10 and 100 miles a week, individual runners of different abilities should be able to find an optimal, adaptive mileage level. That level, whatever it ends up being, will become their training base.

The Long, Slow Training Rationale

A training base is essentially the duration of weekly running at mild-to-light exertion. Unfortunately, the running culture in America tends to overlook light-exertion running as a relatively ineffective way to build racing ability. We are always tempted to train specifically, especially with a goal-race imminent. Besides, the argument goes, how much stamina do we need to finish a 5K?

Clearly, if finishing a race were your goal, you would need less stamina for a 5K than a marathon. If *racing* is your goal, however, then there is no difference in the base required to maximize your ability for a long race or a short one. Whether you are training for the mile or the marathon, being adapted to 100-mile training weeks is better than being adapted to 30-mile training weeks. Arthur Lydiard's New Zealand runners proved this principle years ago.

I'm not suggesting that you personally aim for 100-mile training weeks. I'm simply saying that, when it comes to sustaining that much mileage, you would need an enormous amount of running energy. The goal is to use this energy to build the capacity for shorter, faster workouts and, ultimately, faster races. Nor am I suggesting that you skip steady-state running by focusing on mild or light exertion exclusively.

However, when you consider steady-state running to be your base, you necessarily limit the duration of that base. Since steady state is a higher level than mild and light exertion, you simply can't run as long at steady state as you can at those lower levels. And while intensity is a major adaptive stimulus, *duration* adds its own adaptive dimension.

Of course, if you only have a few hours to train each week, it might be better to train at steady state. When it comes to base mileage, however, the object is to establish the broadest possible base within a reasonable periodic timeframe.

The Step-by-Step Building Process

Several times in this book, I've pointed out the difficulty of establishing a new workout regimen. This is one of the persistent training problems. The key to solving it is to establish a set of workouts that you are passably able to do.

WEEKLY MILEAGE

It's amazing how much ego can be involved with weekly mileage, and how some people resist cutting back on their hard-won gains. When I was in college, I always counted my mileage but I never obsessed about it. When my coach gave me a workout regimen, I ran the workouts, even if it meant cutting back on mileage. Later, on my own, I wasn't so amenable to cutting back, and I hurt myself trying to combine hills and intervals with high mileage.

I had seen runners doing hills and intervals with more mileage than I was running, and I thought I could run similar regimens, too. It was difficult for me to accept that those guys had cut back from even higher mileage regimens. Finally, I harkened back to the days when I relied on my training base to give me extra energy while I did shorter, faster workouts. As difficult as it had been to build a base of stamina, the benefit of all those miles didn't disappear overnight just because I had reduced my mileage.

Building a training base provides an opportunity to use this principle. Let's suppose that you are currently well-adapted to three 30-minute, light-exertion runs per week. You think you could extend the duration of the 30-minute runs to 60 minutes, and you might be able to extend them to 90 minutes. But you wonder which new workouts would *least* likely saddle you with an adverse shock reaction.

Obviously, 60-minute workouts would shock your system less than 90-minute workouts. (In this example, we will consider duration increments of 30 minutes in order to create sharper contrasts.) The 90-minute alternative may seem more attractive because it's the longest. But, rather than trying initially to run the longest regimen, your objective should be to find a balance between too much effort and too little.

Complicating matters is your desire to increase the frequency of your training. Most good runners train every day, and, in this case, let's say you want to be good. Whichever workout duration you adopt, the crucial issue is whether you are passably able to run that long *every* day. Remember, you are already fully able to run 30 minutes three times a week, but that doesn't mean you can run 60 or 90 minutes once a day, seven days a week, at the passable level.

You could choose to run 60 minutes once a day instead of 90 minutes. But this choice would double the frequency and duration of your workouts, while *quadrupling* the duration of your current weekly regimen. Do you see how this might be a recipe for disaster? If you're smart, you'll start with something closer to what you're already able to do. By running 30-minute workouts once a day, for instance, you'll double the frequency and duration of your weekly training, while maintaining the 30-minute workouts you're used to doing.

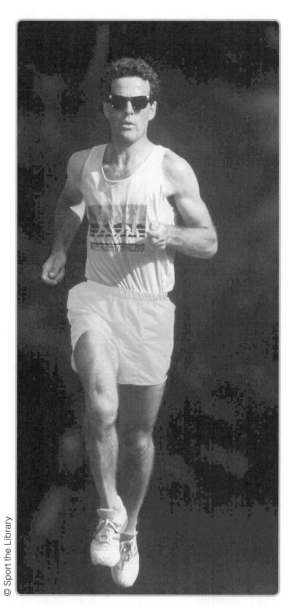

© Sport the Library

The goal of base training is to increase your time on the road at light exertion. Since exertion remains the same, increased energy enables increased duration.

Let's say you try the daily, 30-minute schedule and, to your delight, you are able to sustain it for several weeks without breaking down. In fact, your energy is so good for these easy runs that you decide to up the ante. First, you increase the duration of three of your weekly workouts from 30 to 60 minutes, which also increases their overall effort from easy to moderate. Meanwhile, you maintain easy workouts on the days between the moderate workouts. This moderate-easy-moderate schedule is tougher than the previous easy-easy-easy one, but it's still manageable in terms of energy.

During the next several weeks your muscles are somewhat stiff and sore the day after the moderate workouts. These stress symptoms eventually abate and you discover that your energy is often at the ready-to-run-hard level for your 60-minute moderate workouts. During the next several weeks, therefore, you gradually lengthen the duration of the remaining easy workouts until they, too, are moderate 60-minute efforts. At that point, you realize that you are approaching the limit of your capacity for weekly effort. The easy workouts of the previous schedule allowed you to recover to the point of readiness. But the new regimen consists of daily moderate workouts, and you never feel ready-to-run-hard for any of them.

After several weeks, it becomes apparent that your energy is just barely holding up. You are passably able to maintain your weekly regimen, but you sense that you would break down immediately if you were to run any longer or any faster. The only way you've been able to sustain the moderate/lazy training load is by placing a strict limit on your heart rate. Nonetheless, you decide to maintain this daily, moderate/lazy schedule because your experience indicates it's both optimal and sustainable.

At this point, you've established your training base. It could have been shorter, less frequent, and less arduous, but it couldn't have been harder without courting disaster. What happens next depends on your willingness to be consistent. If you maintain this training load, you will eventually consolidate your base through continued adaptive training.

Sharpening and Peaking

The logic of progressive adaptation demands that you decrease duration whenever you increase exertion. It's better in the context of progressive training to give up some weekly mileage and use the resultant extra energy to build new, more race-specific abilities. Thus, in order to gain ability you have to give it up.

The process of running shorter, faster workouts is called sharpening. Done correctly, the energy you save by running shorter is applied to running at a higher exertion level. In this way you don't overtrain because your workout effort remains at an optimal level. The problem is to know when you've balanced increases in exertion with decreases in duration. That's the subject of the next section.

Starting at the Passably Able Level

The process of transitioning from base training to sharpening always involves the introduction of a new workout. In fact, any time you restructure the exertion of a workout, you create a new workout. Even if you are introducing the same workout you did last year, your body perceives it as a relatively new workout that initiates a new cycle of shock, adaptation, and exhaustion.

Let's say that you are currently adapted to a weekly schedule that includes a 90-minute hard/ready workout. You've been running this workout at light exertion and now you plan to run it faster. A faster workout could build a more race-specific ability, but it could also end up being too hard for your capacity. In setting up the new workout, your primary objective is to be *passably able* to do it.

You think you can balance the faster intervals with a shorter, 70-minute duration, but your exertion for the intervals will still determine how effectively you do the workout. It's always tempting with a new workout to try to impress yourself or your friends with a fast pace. Ironically, the more impressive your pace the more ineffective the workout (see figure 6.1).

Within the zone of ineffectiveness is a stress threshold, which if violated could lead to colds, injuries, and a forced layoff. You won't always be able to tell during a workout that these symptoms are about to hit. Rather, it's usually the next day when you discover the repercussions of overtraining.

If an injury knocks you out for a week, perhaps you'll come back wiser. Meanwhile, the goal of any training period is to be fully able to do your workouts at

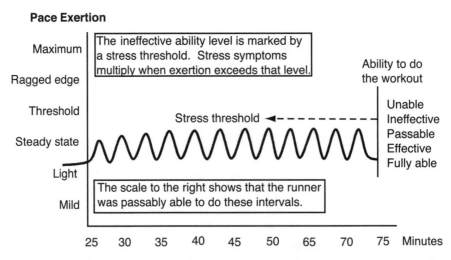

Figure 6.1   The interval portion of this workout is in the steady state range (on the pace exertion scale). At that level you would be "passably able" to do the workout (as indicated by the ability scale on the right). If you were to run the intervals at the threshold level of exertion, you would not only be ineffectively able to do the workout, but you would also surpass a stress threshold, which would likely result in a major setback.

the end of the period. Since you can't adapt until you've established a workout, it's okay to be passably able to do it at the outset. Your starting point is not as important as your ending point.

Stimulating Adaptive Progress

Assuming you've established a new workout, the next objective is to stimulate adaptive progress. In this regard, some runners believe in deliberately increasing their pace to stimulate adaptation. This will work provided that increases in pace correspond to concurrent increases in capacity. Once pace outstrips capacity, exertion rises to spur further increments in pace.

Whenever you increase exertion, you change the established structure of a workout, thereby throwing yourself into shock again. You don't have to increase the exertion of a workout in order to stimulate adaptation. The exertion inherent in a once established workout is sufficient stimulus for adaptation. Until adaptation runs its course, all you need to stimulate further adaptation is to repeat the workout at the established level.

The adaptive results you are looking for depend on your ability-building purpose. When you are building tempo, for instance, the object of adaptation is a faster pace. But getting faster during a training period isn't always what you want. As you adapt to a base-building regimen, for example, some or all of your workouts should get longer, instead of faster. And when you are building power with hills, the adaptive goal is a more vigorous running motion, which doesn't have to involve a faster pace (see table 6.1). If you are fortunate enough to adapt to a workout, that adaptation should manifest itself according to your ability-building purpose. If your purpose is to build stamina, adaptation should manifest itself as an increase in workout duration because that's the purpose of a stamina workout. Tempo, speed, and endurance are race-specific abilities and they should be manifested by a faster pace.

The bottom line? Improved performance should never occur without a concurrent increase in your capacity for exertion. There are only three training variables: effort, capacity, and performance. When it comes to running faster intervals from week to week, your heart rate will remain the same as your capacity expands.

TABLE 6.1   Manifesting Adaptation by Ability-Building Purpose

Purpose	Adaptation manifested as
Stamina	Longer runs at the same mild- to light-exertion heart rate
Power	A more vigorous motion at the same targeted heart rate
Tempo	A faster pace at the same targeted heart rate
Speed	A faster pace at the same targeted heart rate
Endurance	A faster pace at the same targeted heart rate

Aiming at Peak Proficiency

Having developed stamina, power, and tempo during your initial training periods, you have speed and endurance to develop during the peaking period before a goal-race. By radically reducing your training base, you not only find the energy to run at a higher level of exertion, but you will now have abundant energy for all your workouts.

Your energy should be tremendous during the peaking process. It can be difficult psychologically with so much energy to keep from racing your workouts, but the goal is to have abundant energy for the real races. So keep your speed and endurance workouts sharp, but not so long that you need more than 36 hours to recover from them.

At this point, it's fair to ask whether you will jeopardize your racing capacity by giving up your base abilities. In the long term of several months or more, you will certainly jeopardize your ability to race. In the short term of six weeks or so, however, the minimal training of a peaking schedule will see you through until you've raced to your heart's content and it's time to build a base again. Meanwhile, it might help to put peak training in perspective.

A peak is the point of highest proficiency during a training period. By this definition, you can peak during any training period as you become fully able to do your workouts. From the standpoint of performance, it's always best to race at the point of peak proficiency. By tapering you can boost your energy for a race and perform quite well, even though you're in the throes of hard training, and even though you still haven't peaked with a full complement of racing abilities.

Since it's difficult to build all five abilities at once, you have to focus on one set of workouts, and then set them aside to focus on another. By this process, periodic training builds a hierarchy of complementary abilities. Stamina, the base ability, complements power by giving you the energy to build that ability. Similarly, power gives you the muscle strength to take longer strides while you train for tempo. Endurance then consolidates tempo training by giving you the ability to sustain your racing tempo. Finally, speed, the icing on the cake, augments your ability to endure intense race exertion.

Building one ability serves to build another, with the base abilities of stamina, power, and tempo dissipating as you decrease the frequency of those workouts late in a training program. The time frame for these periods is ultimately up to you, but I think of a training program as lasting a year. According to this schedule, base building and sharpening take roughly eight months, leaving about 18 weeks to peak, race, and recover.

Programmatic peaking occurs in context with a metacycle, which is super-imposed upon the entire training program (see figure 6.2). A metacycle develops according to the programmatic progression: base building, sharpening, peaking,

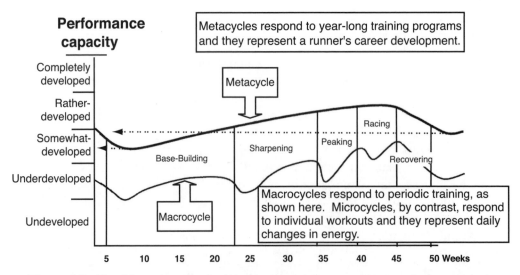

Figure 6.2 The 52-week cycle depicted here could respond to one of many annual training programs that slowly elevate your performance capacity to the completely developed level. The dotted, horizontal arrows indicate a slight gain in capacity from the beginning of this metacycle to the beginning of the next.

racing, and recovering. Ideally, each metacycle peaks during its planned racing period and on the day you want to exert a best effort.

During the peaking process, your performance capacity is like a house of cards. It's mostly held up by adaptation that occurred during the base training and sharpening periods. Performance capacity begins to level off during the peaking and racing periods, and eventually it collapses as your energy reserves become depleted with lots of racing and little training. In this sense, peaking is the final phase of training in which you extend the tapering process so you can be at your best on the day of a goal-event.

The important thing is to see your program as divided naturally, rationally, and holistically into periods lasting about a year. The constant, annual rhythm of programmatic training and racing is what develops your performance capacity in the long term of 5 to 10 years.

The developmental goal is to be a little stronger each year when you come around to building the same set of abilities. In this regard, the constancy of programmatic training is crucial. And, of course, injury, illness, and exhaustion are the bane of long-term, cyclic adaptation.

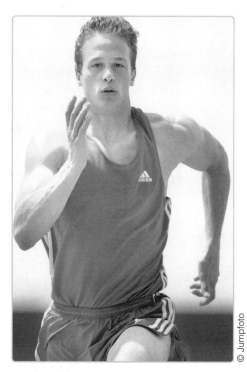

You'll know you are at peak performance capacity when you are fully able to do your workouts.

Tapering and Recovering

The discipline of racing during hard training periods requires tapering before the event. It's especially important to taper before very hard/eager races. You can't expect to bring your energy up to eager with the usual 48- to 60-hour recovery period after a hard workout.

Nor can you prepare your mind for the rigors of a *very* hard effort by sharing your mental focus with hard training efforts. Even a hard/ready workout requires a certain amount of mental preparation. You can't simply walk out the door and perform at the hard/ready level without envisioning the workout, intending certain outcomes, and gathering yourself for the effort.

You must appreciate, therefore, that a very hard/eager racing effort is in a completely different league from normal hard training. With the big races, it's common to begin the focusing process about two weeks before the event. Once this process begins, your mind will withhold psychic energy from your training in an unconscious attempt to gather its resources for the coming effort. As a result, you could have the disconcerting feeling of losing your energy and your ability in the last 10 days.

You must be aware of this gathering syndrome and taper your training so you don't inadvertently exhaust yourself. The bigger the event psychologically, the more you'll have to taper in order to keep from overtraining. In the last couple of weeks before a big race, all bets are off when it comes to normal training and recovery processes. Yet, since it's rare to feel that we've trained enough, it's easy to convince ourselves that we need that one last workout. Unfortunately, that workout isn't the same as the workouts in a normal training week. Your energy won't be as good, and neither will your recoveries.

It's up to you to experiment with different tapering patterns to see what works best in different circumstances. If you race during a base-building or sharpening period, proper tapering could take a week or two. Except for the race itself, such a dearth of training could detract from ability-building processes. Although the adaptive value of a very hard/eager race is considerable, it doesn't necessarily compensate for several missed hard/ready workouts. Notwithstanding this training shortfall, it's okay to race as frequently as once every three or four weeks.

Some athletes try to "train through" a race by skimping on their taper and their recovery. But the arbiter is still your experience of energy, and something is wrong when you don't have enough of it to train or race effectively. You should strive to do the right things in your training, so you can build the discipline to do exactly what you intend in your races.

Postrace Danger Points

Some runners say they need a day of recovery for every all-out racing mile. It's more accurate to say they need one day of recovery for every all-out/*eager* racing mile. There's a big difference between running all-out/eager and all-out/ready. Being eager creates a much greater capacity for exertion and a correspondingly faster performance.

The amount of recovery time you'll need after a race depends on the size of the effort, the size of your capacity and the number of racing miles. Since this book is about 5K and 10K racing, we don't have to be concerned with longer racing distances, which generally require longer recoveries. Rather, 5K and 10K races are short enough that you can expect to recover from them within a week, even when you've run all-out/eager.

Nonetheless, there is a definite discipline to the recovery process following a race. One of the biggest mistakes you can make is to jam a hard workout into a racing recovery period. Typically, you'll run a 5K and feel like you are ready to run hard the next day. It's common to have energy left over from a short race like the 5K and from the tapering prior to the race. But the danger is from the increased risk of injury in the 24 hours after a sharp racing effort.

BUILDING MILEAGE

Most of us know the formulas for extending mileage in certain small and regular increments. It makes sense to increase a training load in this way, especially when you are already pushing the envelope of available energy for a long run or a long weekly regimen. These formulas don't necessarily apply, however, when athletes are building mileage from scratch and they have energy to spare.

In my training program for the Honolulu Marathon, for example, my athletes pay me to train them three times a week for 14 weeks. During the first three weeks of the training, I regularly increase the duration of their long runs from a starting level of 60 minutes to two hours. Often, the longest runs these athletes have done prior to entering the program were about 30 minutes. They can increase their time on the road this rapidly only because they keep their exertion at the mild-to-light level, using noticeable fatigue as an indication that they've reached their duration limit.

During the Honolulu Marathon training, novice runners keep the pace of a group leader who knows how to hold the pace back to mild exertion in the early going. If you don't have someone to set the pace for you, you may have to use a heart rate monitor to regulate your pace. Once you know your maximum heart rate, mild and light exertion will be 50 to 59% and 60 to 69% of maximum, respectively. Depending on your maximum, however, those combined levels could be 40 beats per minute wide. It's okay to target your exertion anywhere within that range, but I recommend starting at the low end and bringing your heart rate up gradually as your energy develops within a workout

It's common for leftover hormonal energy to linger for 24 hours after a race. Some hormones gear your body up for exertion while others are natural pain killers. Such hormones have a life cycle that can overlap postrace training, but those hormones dissipate eventually. Thus the second day after a race is likely to be the worst in terms of energy and inflammation. This low-energy and potential-injury syndrome is exacerbated by hard training immediately after a race. No matter how you feel the day after a race, you should refrain from hard training in anticipation of the inevitable postrace low.

The next danger point occurs several days after a race when it's common to feel prematurely recovered. You could, for instance, feel a false sense of energy on Wednesday or Thursday after a Sunday race. Typically, you will start a workout feeling ready, and discover about halfway through that you have far less energy than you thought. You'd be wise at that point to back off immediately, and wiser still to schedule moderate workouts in the week following a difficult race.

Programmatic Recovery Periods

Peaking and racing periods are restful enough that we tend to forget what "real" training is about. Yet, within a week of running a goal-race you could be back to the daily grind of base training and, before you know it, you're locked into the discipline of a new training schedule, despite nagging injuries and a running spirit that needs a rest.

Ambitious personalities find it difficult, if not impossible, to do nothing but easy training. It seems such a waste of time. Yet, I've seen good runners turn pale and haggard from too much hard training. They were exhausted and refused to acknowledge it. Some contracted serious illnesses that took them permanently out of the competitive game. In my case, experience has taught me the value of taking time off. Now, recovery is just another necessary "training" period, scheduled as a matter of course.

You should think about what you most need from a recovery period and schedule your workouts accordingly. Obviously, total exhaustion and major injury should be treated differently from less problematic conditions. In the final analysis,

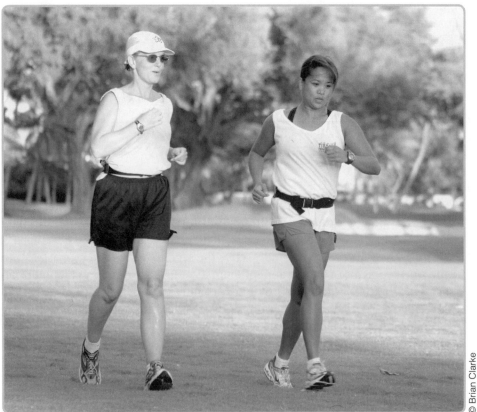

© Brian Clarke

The final phase of a training program is a period of recovery when it's okay to do only easy workouts.

we must want to be in the game at all levels of our being. If we don't enjoy our training and racing, then we'll eventually find a way to take ourselves out of it, accidentally or on purpose.

Thus, it's a good idea to deliberately take time off once a year to bring your competitive being into balance. Just think of it as a vacation from timed workouts on measured courses, carrying a heart rate monitor and running hard workouts. Try running for the pure enjoyment of it, at least until your ambition coalesces around a new training plan.

Postprogram Planning and Review

Being in recovery mode is an opportunity to reflect on the past year and to plan for the year to come. There is always something to learn from the recent campaign, and there is always some new idea to apply to the next one. Thus, I find myself ruminating about the way the past year developed.

Did I get sick, injured, or exhausted? How come? What can I do differently to avoid those problems next time? Did I have mostly great races or were some of them only fair? How come? What did I do that was right and what can I do better next time? In thinking about reasons things went wrong, you must be aware of where you locate causal factors.

It's not enough to say the weather, the course, or our competitors were the reasons we didn't perform well. If causes are outside of us, then we are not taking responsibility for our experience. We must be accountable for every problem that occurred. Otherwise, we give up our personal power to improve our training and racing and, in the process, we doom ourselves to repeating the same negative experiences.

It usually takes me a couple of years after a comeback to see realistic possibilities for progressive training and racing. Only after those initial programmatic experiences do I have a knowledge base upon which I can build a realistic program. Having a coach who knows the game and has a good sense of what you can handle could put you ahead on the learning curve. Otherwise, you are on your own to muddle through, using your wits and intelligence to think about how you might solve the recurring training and racing problems.

Competitive running isn't an easy game to master. It's about lifting your ability to new developmental levels. It's about learning from your experience and honing workouts and time frames to be more effective adaptive stimuli. Ultimately, it's about your storied journey toward mastery in the game of running.

Taking the Next Step

This chapter has anticipated the next two by considering some issues related to programmatic training. This last section will aim you in the direction of setting up a training program in preparation for a goal-race. There are several interrelated issues to consider as you begin tailoring a training program to suit your needs and time frame.

How many weeks will it take to introduce and establish a new workout? This depends on the number of steps you'll need to introduce the new workout without hurting yourself initially. If your old and new workouts are similar in structure, you can introduce a new workout in relatively little time, say, a couple of weeks. Otherwise, it could take you a month to make the necessary steps without becoming sick or injured.

How many new workouts do you plan to introduce? A full complement of new workouts could represent a major shock to your system, which could increase the time you'll need to establish the regimen. Four to six weeks is not a long time to make this initial adjustment. And at that point you will have only established the regimen.

Once you've established a new workout, how many weeks will you need to adapt to it? You may see some progress within several weeks, but the real issue is the amount of time it will take to become fully able to do the workout, assuming you are only passably able to do it once it's established. Six weeks is not a long time to adapt to a new workout or a new training regimen.

Once you've milked a workout for maximum gains in proficiency, how much time remains before your goal-race? Do you have enough time to reestablish a new workout regimen *and* gain proficiency from it? If so, what new workouts will take the place of your recent regimen? Here, you must answer the same questions you just answered for the last set of workouts. The next chapter will augment your understanding of how to construct a training program by giving you ideas for structuring individual ability-building workouts.

CHAPTER 7

Designing Workouts to Build Ability

They say that legendary football coach Vince Lombardi could speak for hours about one end-run play in his team's playbook. I don't mean to put myself in Lombardi's Super Bowl winning class, but I do know about the workouts in my repertoire. This chapter describes a number of those ability-building workouts. You can use these descriptions as models for workouts during your 5K or 10K training. Or you can think about your own workouts from my perspective to see how you might adjust your training given new ideas.

Most of the workouts I'll describe in this chapter have an upper heart rate limit, which is presented as a percent of your maximum heart rate. I described a way of measuring your maximum heart rate in chapter 1. You may want to run that workout to measure your maximum before you try to run the workouts described here. Running any of these workouts correctly assumes that you are using a heart rate monitor to establish narrow target heart rate zones.

Similarly, you should know your capacity for exertion, whether high, medium, or low. I gave you a series of questions to assess your capacity in chapters 1 and 4. If you haven't already answered those questions, you should do so before trying these workouts. Knowing your capacity will enable you to adjust the workouts so you don't inadvertently overtrain.

Finally, you should make a distinction between capacity for exertion and your current performance capacity for the 5K and 10K. Performance capacity is your ability to perform a race in minutes. Table 7.1 will help you estimate your performance capacity so you can develop workouts appropriate to your ability.

TABLE 7.1   Performance Capacity Based on 5K and 10K Times

Ability	5K	10K
Elite runner 1	12:45 to 14:30	26:00 to 30:00
Elite runner 2	14:31 to 17:20	30:01 to 36:00
Competitive runner 1	17:21 to 23:30	36:01 to 49:00
Competitive runner 2	23:31 to 30:00	49:01 to 62:00
Recreational runner	30:01 to 35:00	62:01 to 74:00

Base Workouts

A training base is the sustainable duration of weekly running. The more hours you can run without crashing, the broader your base. This simple concept also applies to the duration of individual workouts, including the workouts with which you begin a training program. Those workouts are your base workouts.

There are three types of base workout: 1) recovery runs that remain relatively short and slow while contributing to your base of stamina; 2) a designated long run that grows in duration as your stamina increases; and 3) other base workouts that evolve during a training program to build your ability for power, tempo, speed, and endurance.

Depending on the time you have to train and your need to build a training base, all of your workouts could be stamina runs during a base-building period. Eventually, however, some workouts will become increasingly race-specific. In this section, I'm mostly concerned about issues related to the workout you designate to build your ability for long, slow running. How long should that workout be at the beginning, middle, and end of the program? And how frequently should you run it?

The most important issue to decide is your starting duration. In table 7.2, I've presented nine duration guidelines for introducing long-run workout duration, based on whether your capacity is high, medium, or low, and whether you want the workout to be hard or moderate.

TABLE 7.2   Duration Guidelines for Introducing a Stamina Workout

Capacity	Hard/Ready	Moderate/Ready	Moderate/Lazy
High	90 min	80 min	70 min
Medium	80 min	70 min	60 min
Low	70 min	60 min	50 min

Suppose you want to do a hard/ready workout and you have medium capacity, as determined by the answers you gave in chapters 1 and 4. According to table 7.2, you would start with an 80-minute run. Theoretically, the high-capacity, 90-minute option would be too long and the low-capacity, 70-minute option would be too short. But, of course, your workout effort isn't based only on duration but also on your average level of exertion during the workout.

Ultimately, the duration of a workout should depend on your experience of effort and fatigue, as well as the time you need to recover from it. You shouldn't run a two-hour workout merely because you think two hours is better than one. Two hours is not better than one if you become sick, injured, or exhausted trying to do two-hour workouts. Remember, you have a weekly schedule to uphold. If you are scheduled for a hard/ready long run, your workout effort has to fit within that effort/energy context in order to maintain adaptive processes.

Adaptation produces extra energy, which you can use to increase the duration of your long runs. As long as you feel this added energy on a long run, it's okay to run longer. In the process, adaptation is enhanced by doing a long run at least once a week. Although duration and intensity are major adaptive stimuli, frequency adds its own adaptive dimension. The more frequently you do a workout, the more powerful the adaptive stimulus. Since stamina is the base ability, the earlier you are in a program, the more frequently you should train for stamina.

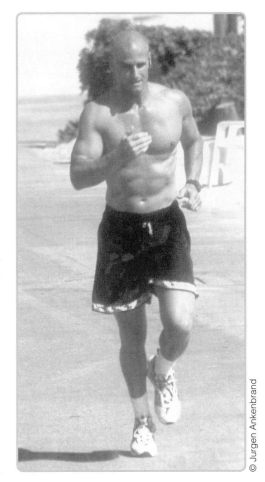

© Jurgen Ankenbrand

Once the sharpening and peaking periods begin, however, you should phase your long runs out by running them on a progressively less frequent basis. During the last month or two before your goal-race, it's okay to run long as little as once every two or three weeks. As you decrease the frequency of a long run, you'll forget how to run it. It makes sense, therefore, to shorten its duration so you don't do something you've forgotten how to do, which is run for a long time. As long as you can maintain some minimal mental and physical contact with running long, however, it will be easier to pick up your long runs when you start building a base again after your current training program.

The following workout description is intended to assist you with planning and establishing a stamina workout. The actual

Workout duration should be a function of balancing a limited amount of available energy with the exertion necessary to practice a racing ability.

DESIGNATED STAMINA WORKOUT

Given the projected starting duration of a new long run (see table 7.2), plan how you will gradually establish the workout over several weeks by adding duration from your current to the projected level. Develop an out-and-back or loop course suited to your capacity and your scheduled workout effort. Begin each workout by warming up at mild exertion for at least 30 to 60 minutes. You may increase your exertion level during the workout as long as you don't exceed the light-exertion limit (69 percent of maximum) and you don't run harder than scheduled. Develop a set of target heart rate zones for the warm-up, the middle, and the ending sections of the run.

The terrain of a long-run course can vary from flat to hilly. It follows that the same workout can have two ability-building purposes: stamina and power. Since your primary purpose is building stamina, however, you have to run the hills at mild to light exertion, which means running them at a slower pace than you would at the same heart rate on level ground.

exertion structure of the workout depends on three factors: 1) the difficulty of the workout, as you have scheduled it into a week of training; 2) your capacity for long-run exertion, as based on your recent training; and 3) your performance capacity, as based on your performance in a recent 5K or 10K race.

There are several course configurations for a stamina run.

< **Out-and-Back**. Start in one place, go out on a course to a turn-around point, and come back the same way you went out. Usually, you'll come back a little faster than you went out because you are warmed up and running at a slightly higher level of exertion. Coming back at a slower pace usually means you went out too fast and became prematurely fatigued.

< **Multiple Loops.** A multiple loop course allows you to stay close to your start/finish point, which gives you the flexibility of stopping soon after reaching your target level of fatigue. In order to add variety to the course, you can run two loops or even several loops, with your start/finish point at or near the intersection of the loops. A loop course gives you the possible convenience of a restroom and an aid station on every loop.

< **One Big Loop.** A big loop offers the advantage of ranging widely, often through a variety of interesting locations and terrain. Big loops can be challeng-

ing, however, because, like the out-and-back course, you can be far from home at certain points. The challenge is to judge your energy correctly early in the run so you get back without overextending yourself. If you sense inadequate energy early in the run, it's up to you to take a shortcut so your workout effort suits your energy.

< **Discovery Run.** This sort of "course" begins with a starting point and a time limit for the workout, say, two hours. As you run, you discover the course in the moment by serendipity and inspiration, and according to your energy. This sort of run is fun to do at the start of a training period when you are, in fact, deciding what your long-run course will be, once established.

Recovery Workouts

Recovery runs are a special case of stamina training. By adding light-exertion recovery training to your major workout regimen, you can double your weekly mileage and significantly increase the stimulus for building stamina.

If you've never taken the time to build your capacity in this way, you might be surprised at the amount of stamina you can build. It takes a lot of energy to run every day, and much more energy to do the same recovery run twice a day. But if you maintain the adaptive stimulus, you could provide yourself with more energy than you've ever had for running.

Depending on how much energy you have left over after running the major workouts on your weekly schedule, you can run as many recovery runs as you want. The downside to so much running is the constant heavy-legged, logy feeling of having little energy between your major workouts. Your stride loses its snap, and with it goes any semblance of speed you may have had only weeks before. As your fatigue continues, you wonder whether you are doing irreparable damage to your ability to run fast.

It takes courage, patience, and discipline to run so slowly and so often. With double workouts, it seems like you hardly have time for life outside of running workouts and changing clothes. Even the discipline of running only once a day can be demanding. Many athletes are accustomed to taking days off to restore their energy. Forty-eight hours without running is normal for them; taking only 12 hours off is beyond their comprehension. Once adapted to a double workout regimen, however, even 36 hours seems like a long time to rest.

You cannot build your ability unless you maintain an adaptive stimulus. You are doomed if you have a life that interferes with the discipline of running workouts. It doesn't matter what your regimen is, you've got to maintain the discipline. Sometimes that means being more faithful to your workout schedule than to work and family. Few people outside of school have the opportunity to commit themselves to such a training regimen.

I'm not saying that every athlete has to run twice a day. In this book, I assume you either have the opportunity and the capacity to run twice a day, or you don't.

Some athletes are better off with a regimen that allows them to take days off. In any case, whatever your weekly regimen, you've got to commit yourself to following through.

Tempo Workouts

Tempo is the ability to run comfortably at race pace. Being comfortable implies that you feel little or no sense of race-specific intensity. You should keep this idea firmly in mind as you train for tempo as opposed to speed and endurance, which are completely different abilities that require higher levels of race-specific intensity.

This section focuses on two types of tempo training: steady state and pace specific. Here, pace-specific tempo refers to the way your pace feels while you are running the first half of a goal-race. Since your tempo for the 5K and 10K can be rapid and pressing, pace-specific tempo intervals have to be short enough to avoid the sort of discomfort you can expect during the second half of your goal-race.

By contrast, steady-state tempo intervals are generally longer and slower than pace-specific tempo intervals. Well-trained athletes can usually maintain exertion at the quick and relaxed steady-state level for at least several minutes without discomfort. The key to a steady-state interval workout is to make the intervals slow enough that your breathing remains inaudible, despite their relatively long duration. Of course, you may hear yourself as you inhale and exhale, but someone running beside you would only hear occasional huffs in your conversation.

Steady-State Tempo Runs

I think of steady-state tempo training as forming a transition between light-exertion long runs and pace-specific tempo workouts. A steady-state tempo workout could take about 70 to 80 minutes, including warm-up, tempo intervals, rest intervals, and cool-down (see the following workout description).

If you've previously built a base workout totaling at least 90 to 100 minutes of light-exertion running, you shouldn't have a problem adjusting to a steady-state interval workout totaling 70 to 80 minutes. You may still be doing long, slow workouts in other workout time slots, but the particular long, slow workout with which you began this tempo progression has been morphed into a completely different ability-building structure.

The purpose of the new workout is to increase your tempo ability. It isn't necessarily the pace-specific tempo of the 5K or 10K, but it could qualify as tempo for a longer race. And it's definitely quicker than the light-exertion stamina runs from which it originated. In fact, if you are a jogger level athlete, a quick, relaxed tempo could qualify as pace-specific for the 10K, because the duration of your race is long enough to force you to slow down to this steady-state level.

STEADY-STATE TEMPO INTERVALS

1. Warm up for 15 minutes at mild-to-light exertion.
2. On a running track or a measured grassy course (see page 104), do a set of quick and relaxed, 5- to 7-minute intervals, jogging very slowly without stopping for 75 seconds between intervals. Target your heart rate in a narrow range of five beats per minute, not to exceed the following: elite runners 76 percent of maximum, competitive runners 74 percent, and recreational runners 72 percent. Depending on your scheduled level of workout effort, build from six to eight intervals (hard workout) or three to five intervals (moderate workout) during the first three weeks.
3. Cool down for 5 minutes at light-to-mild exertion.

Ideally, a new tempo workout will be moderately challenging, but not impossible to do. You should carry a stopwatch and heart rate monitor in your hand for referencing your pace and heart rate. But the most important information during the process of establishing the workout is the biofeedback you receive about holding a quick, relaxed tempo. Quick is between slow and rapid; relaxed is between held back and pressed. These are descriptions of the way exertion feels while you are running. You must pay attention to your effort in order to make these distinctions.

The effort volume for a steady-state tempo workout can be daunting. It's up to you to choose a way to gradually increase its volume during several workouts. You could abbreviate the number of intervals during the first few workouts, as I've suggested in the workout description. Or you could do the full number of intervals at either a lower target heart rate or half the tempo interval distance. With the first workout under your belt, you can increase your heart rate or the distance of the interval during subsequent workouts, until you are doing the whole workout at the scheduled level.

You must adopt a disciplined approach to doing a base-interval workout. You should be consistently ready for the workout, and you should run only your scheduled level of workout difficulty, whether moderate or hard. Somehow you've got to recognize the point to end the workout, which depends on recognizing a certain level of fatigue. When you are running a hard workout, for instance, you'll aim for noticeable and significant fatigue. When you are running a moderate workout you'll aim for appreciable but minor fatigue.

As you become fatigued during a hard workout, you'll have difficulty keeping your heart rate from rising above your target zone. It could be that you've increased your pace, but, if your pace is the same as earlier, then you've reached your workout limit and it's time to stop, regardless of the number of intervals you may have done. Assuming you're becoming too fatigued and too inefficient to continue at an adaptive level, quitting is more important than running a certain quota of intervals.

Here's another trick for recognizing noticeable fatigue. You're there when you discover you've slowed down during an interval in which you've maintained your usual target heart rate. Obviously, you'll need a target heart rate and you'll have to pay attention to your times, while keeping yourself within a target zone. That's all part of the discipline of doing any interval workout, including pace-specific interval workouts.

Pace-Specific Tempo Training

Once you've adapted to a steady-state interval workout, you should restructure that workout, creating a shorter, faster, race-specific interval workout. The purpose of this workout will be to build pace-specific tempo for the 5K or 10K you aim to run later in the program.

Pace-specific tempo training is different from the steady-state tempo training I described earlier, despite the fact that pace-specific intervals are also usually run at steady state. Pace-specific tempo training duplicates the feeling of your current racing pace, especially the comfortable, light, and easy feeling of the first half of a race when you are not yet fatigued and pushing to sustain the pace.

Training exactly at race pace is less important than recognizing the way race pace feels and being able to duplicate that feeling in a workout. During a training run, your pace will probably be slower than race pace because your energy is usually not as good, so your steps are not as long. But your training pace can nonetheless feel like race pace because you are taking about the same number of steps per minute, and pushing about as hard, too.

Knowing your current race pace is a key ingredient in this equation. You should have an idea of how fast you can run 5K or 10K. The best way to reveal your current performance capacity is to step into a race and run it for time. It doesn't matter that you didn't run a best effort; leave that for your goal-race. All you need is an approximation of your current ability. Once you have a finish time for a race, you can correctly estimate your average pace in minutes per mile. This is as fast as you should run during your pace-specific tempo training.

I personally run my tempo intervals about 9 to 11 percent slower than my current race pace. That training pace feels most like racing tempo to me, especially when my energy is only ample instead of abundant. Some athletes think that running slower than race pace feels too slow, usually because their race pace doesn't represent a best racing effort. In any case, a pace-specific tempo interval should feel somewhat slow. None of the intervals in a pace-specific tempo work-

PACE-SPECIFIC TEMPO WORKOUT.

1. Warm up for 15 minutes at mild-to-light exertion.
2. Run a series of tempo intervals with a 60-second rest jog between each interval. Do not exceed 20 intervals for the 10K and 25 intervals for the 5K.

Interval duration should be 50 to 70 seconds for the 5K and 90 to 130 seconds for the 10K. Establish a constant interval distance according to these times during the first week, and, by the third week, establish a narrow target heart rate range of five beats per minute not to exceed the following: elite runners 79 percent of maximum, competitive runners 77 percent, and recreational runners 75 percent. If you are uncertain of your maximum heart rate, aim for a pace that's about 10 percent slower than your current race pace, and do not run faster than your current 5K or 10K race pace during the workout.

out should feel faster than race pace, because it's difficult to sustain adequate training volume at that pace without overtraining.

Pace-specific adaptation derives from the total duration of tempo running. There are several reasons to structure workouts with tempo intervals that amount to a significant proportion of your goal-race distance. First, by repeating high-volume tempo workouts, you'll develop the capacity to run the first half of your race at a comfortable racing tempo. You'll also develop the ability to pace yourself correctly for the whole race. After running hundreds of tempo intervals, you'll know intuitively at the start of a race whether your tempo is too fast, too slow, or just right to finish without crashing.

There are several factors to keep in mind as you run a pace-specific tempo workout including rest, venues, and injuries. First, you should not hear your breathing during these intervals. Even if the workout description calls for your heart rate to rise to the elite level, 79 percent of maximum is still a little lower than the audible-breathing threshold of 80. Second, the distance/duration of the tempo interval cannot be so short that you find yourself running faster than your current race pace.

You may play with the duration of the tempo intervals suggested in the workout description on this page until you are running at or a little slower than your current race pace, but the heart rate limit is more important than your pace. And when it comes to breathing, don't breathe audibly.

> **Rest intervals.** Many beginner athletes feel that running a tempo interval gives them the right to stand around during the rest break. Others walk instead of jog. They don't realize that the rest interval should be timed and controlled as assiduously as the tempo interval. Some athletes dilly-dally for two or three minutes between intervals, talking to their friends or getting water. These habits are definitely not part of the intervallic discipline.

The Jeff Galloway system of marathon running calls for intermittent walking, which is a good way of conserving energy during a marathon. Interval training uses the same principle to conserve energy that would be otherwise used with sustained tempo running. In this training system, however, the discipline is to jog very slowly through the entire rest interval. That means you shouldn't walk at all during your rest intervals. At the end of a tempo interval you slow down to a very slow jog, and when it's time to start the next tempo interval you pick up the pace, without stopping or walking.

Some athletes can't abide by the idea of jogging at their slowest pace during the rest interval. They move along at a quick pace that rivals their tempo pace, so they can "maintain a training level." They don't appreciate the discipline of interval training, which includes tempo running alternated with very slow jogging. A very slow jog brings your heart rate down quickly, while keeping you warmed up and ready for the next tempo interval.

> **Interval training venues.** You can run an interval workout on the road, but there are far better places, as the following suggestions indicate.

- **Running track.** A 400-meter running track with a smooth and resilient all-weather surface is a good environment for intervals because you'll know your distance and your pace exactly with every interval. It's beyond the scope of this book to cover all the layout and distance possibilities of various kinds of tracks. The main thing to understand is that distance increases as you run farther from the inner lane, so you should run as close as possible to the inside of the track where your distance will be accurate. Ask the people who maintain the track to explain its features so you know how far you are running.

- **Measured course in a grassy park.** I recommend borrowing or renting a measuring wheel so you can measure various courses in a level, grassy park. As a minimum, you should have a 400-meter or quarter-mile straightaway and an 800-meter or half-mile loop. Thick, soft grass will slow you down a little, but it also minimizes the risk of injury (pounding causes many common running injuries). On a straightaway course, you can take a short recovery jog at each end, running back-and-forth for the tempo interval.

> **Injuries.** Most of the injuries I see as a coach are shoe-related. Inexperienced runners tend to overuse their shoes. Too much wear on the sole or compression in the midsole increases the risk of injury. This is especially true on the track, because many runners use light trainers or racing flats to run their intervals, and

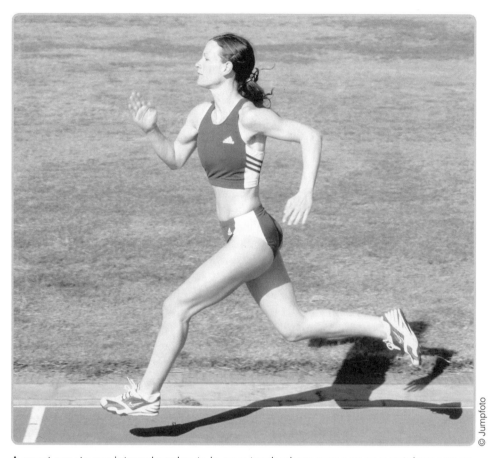

© Jumpfoto

A great way to run interval workouts is on a track where you can accurately measure your distance and pace with every interval.

light-weight shoes wear out much faster than heavier models. I'm not saying which shoes to wear; just be careful. Change your shoes at the first sign of injury.

Interval training is often injurious for several other reasons. First, inexperienced runners equate intervals with words like fast and speed, and they attack their intervals accordingly. Often, there's too big a difference between the pace they are used to running and the pace they think they have to run during an "interval" workout. That's why I've given you heart rate limits for various workouts. Abide by those limits.

> **Other types of pace-specific tempo training.** Endurance training refers to pace-specific tempo intervals that are long enough to match the specific intensity of the second half of your goal-race. Speed intervals are a notch faster than endurance intervals, but, because speed intervals are shorter, your heart rate and your experience of discomfort will be about the same as endurance intervals. Although pace-specific tempo intervals are run at the same tempo as endurance

intervals, tempo intervals are shorter than endurance intervals, and also shorter than steady-state intervals.

Power Workouts

The power workouts in a 5K or 10K program should increase the strength, explosiveness, and reflexivity of your leg muscles and tendons. The large prime-mover muscles on the back of your legs and butt are the main focus of hill training. But your Achilles tendons can also benefit, along with the quadriceps on the front of your upper legs.

Hill training builds the strength for race-specific tempo training. It belongs early in a training program as a prelude to faster running, but some runners put hill training late in a program because they want to be in better shape for hill work, which they consider too difficult for base training. It's only difficult, however, because they run their hills too fast.

Proper hill training is too slow to be placed late in a training program, when most running should be pace-specific. Uphill running shouldn't be pace-specific because it always requires stepping from one elevation to a higher elevation. Depending on the grade of the hill, stepping upward can require significant exertion and muscle strength. Since exertion is the adaptive stimulus, a fast pace in the hills is liable to be much too fast for adaptive purposes.

You should always strive for an uphill pace that's appropriate for your current strength and conditioning. The easiest way to get up a hill is to employ a gliding technique similar to a marathon shuffle on level ground. Your weight will be evenly distributed between the balls of your feet and your heels. There is nothing wrong with that sort of uphill running, as long as the hills aren't so steep that you hurt yourself.

As you progress from the gliding stage, you'll be able to "bounce" uphill on the balls of your feet. On a gradual slope, your heels will kiss the ground; on a steeper hill, they won't touch the ground at all. This bouncing technique involves little or no knee lift, as the motion is mostly from the ankle as you spring off the balls of your forefeet. As you gain muscle strength, you'll be able to take progressively longer, more vigorous bouncing steps at the same target heart rate. The easiest level is called slow bouncing, the next level is quick bouncing, and the third level is exaggerated bouncing.

Exaggerated bouncing is a forward leap or bounding motion off the balls of your feet. Your knees rise in front, and your trailing leg extends behind you. Bounding up short, steep hills may be appropriate for the strongest, fastest runners who have built themselves to the bounding level. But most athletes will never get to this bounding stage of running hills because they are simply unable to sustain a bounding motion without major risk of injury. You may be able to attack a very short hill with a vigorous motion. In general, however, you will be better off using slow or quick bouncing for longer hills. Table 7.3 will get you in the ballpark for adjusting your hill running motion to your ability.

TABLE 7.3   Hill Technique for Different Ability Levels

Ability	Technique	Exertion Target
Recreational runner	Slow glide	Light-to-steady
Competitive runner 2	Slow bouncing	Light-to-steady
Competitive runner 1	Quick bouncing	Steady state
Elite runner 2	Exaggerated bouncing	Steady-to-threshold
Elite runner 1	Bounding	Steady-to-threshold

The best way to introduce muscle strengthening during a base-building period is with long and gentle hills. You don't have to exceed your light-exertion range while doing these hills. You can maintain your target zone for building stamina, albeit at a slower pace than on the flats. I know world-class athletes who walk up steep hills to maintain their target heart rate during a base-building period.

As a next step up from light exertion hill training, you can target steady-state exertion, the heart rate range between 70 and 79 percent of maximum. In establishing a workout at this level, you would be well advised to keep to the lower side of steady state if your hills have been at light exertion thus far.

You should use your heart rate monitor to establish a heart rate limit for running hills, aiming for step-wise increases commensurate with your capacity. The following workout description will get you in the ballpark for establishing a steady-state hill circuit workout.

STEADY-STATE HILL CIRCUIT WORKOUT

Develop a hill circuit or a station course (see below), building the duration of uphill running from 15 percent of total workout time to 20 percent, and then 25 percent during the first three weeks. If 25 percent seems insufficient after the third week, you may increase your hill work to 33 percent of total workout time during the next two weeks. Your heart rate on the uphills should not exceed the following steady-state limits: elite runners 74 percent of maximum, competitive runners 72 percent, and recreational runners 70 percent. You may vary the time of the hill intervals and vary your running motion according to the length of the hill, but use a running motion that's appropriate to your target heart rate and your running capacity. Run at least 15 to 20 minutes at mild-to-light exertion before your first hill interval, and run at least 2 to 3 minutes between hill intervals.

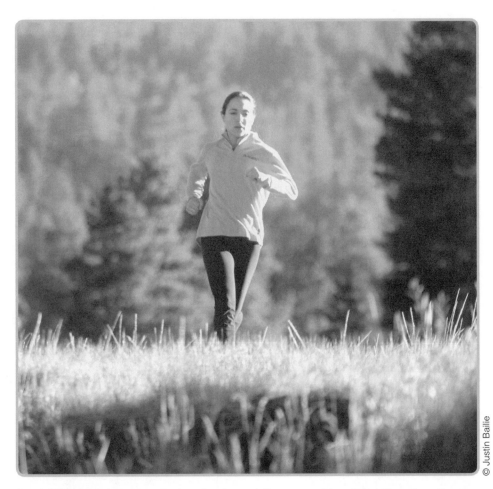

Run hill intervals in a rectangular circuit—uphill on one side, downhill on the other, and flat sections in between.

Unless you're into driving to reach a hilly area, you'll probably have to settle for topographical features available near your home or work. You are looking for moderately challenging hills that are not too steep for your ability.

The standard interval workout in the hills makes use of a rectangular circuit with an uphill on one side, a downhill on the other, and flatter connecting sections. You can also do multiple repetitions of different hills before moving on to another hill. This sort of hill station course may give you more variety than repeating a circuit. You can wander from hill to hill, finding short and steep hills, long and gradual hills, and even an appropriate grassy downhill.

Downhill running builds your ability to take quicker steps. But it can also be injurious because the extreme pounding of your feet against hard pavement during downhill running increases the risk of injury. I instruct my athletes to confine pace-specific downhill running to races only. They are usually rested well enough during a race that downhill running at race pace will not be a big injury risk. If you must practice running downhill, find a course that affords a smooth, grassy, gentle slope. The grass will soften the shock of landing hard and, thereby, lower the injury risk associated with downhill running at a pace-specific tempo.

Having consolidated your ability with hill training, the next step is to phase hills out of your progression while phasing tempo training in. The following transition workout is still moderately long during this process.

TRACK AND HILL INTERVAL WORKOUT

1. Warm up for 15 minutes at mild-to-light exertion on a 400-meter running track.

2. Run a set of pace-specific intervals on the track (4 x 50 seconds for 5K or 4 x 80 seconds for 10K). Don't let your rest interval exceed 60 seconds or drop under 50 seconds. Adjust the duration of the track intervals so you are running your current race pace without audible breathing. Don't exceed the following heart rate limits: elite runners 79 percent of maximum, competitive runners 77 percent, and recreational runners 75 percent. Establish interval distances during the first workout based on the distances you cover as indicated by the above duration instructions. Use a heart rate monitor to pace the intervals according to targets you establish by the second or third workout.

3. Leave the track and run a hill circuit or hill station course (of variable duration up to 60 minutes, depending on your capacity and the scheduled effort of the workout). Reduce the duration of uphill running by 20 percent from your steady-state hill workout and increase the vigor of the hill intervals over a period of three weeks according to the following: Target heart rates of elite runners should not exceed 78 percent of maximum, competitive runners 76 percent, and recreational runners 74 percent. Take enough rest between all hill intervals to bring your exertion down one level. In establishing the length of your hill intervals, run until your heart rate rises above the target level. At that point, you should immediately slow down and take a rest until your heart rate drops a full exertion level and you are ready to start again. As long as you make a distinction between pace-specific training on the flats and hill training that is slower, you should be okay at steady-state exertion, with the usual caveats.

(continued)

Track and Hill Interval Workout *(continued)*

4. Return to the track and run a set of speed-specific intervals (4 × 30 seconds for 5K or 4 × 60 seconds for 10K). Target heart rates for elite runners should not exceed 78 percent of maximum, competitive runners 76 percent, and recreational runners 74 percent. Take enough rest between speed intervals to bring your exertion down one level. The faster pace of a speed interval is related to the shorter time in which you must raise your heart rate to the target limit. Establish interval distances during the first workout based on the distances you cover as indicated by the above duration instructions. Use a heart rate monitor to pace the intervals according to targets you establish by the second or third workout.

5. Cool down at a slow pace for 5 minutes.

Endurance-Speed Workouts

Endurance training is pace-specific tempo running extended for longer intervals. The purpose of endurance training is to build the ability to sustain race-specific intensity. Speed intervals, by contrast, raise intensity to the same race-specific level as the endurance intervals, but they are shorter and faster than endurance intervals. In fact, speed intervals will be the shortest and fastest intervals you ever do.

You shouldn't have to slow down drastically in the last intervals because you went out too fast in the first intervals. Nor should your heart rate rise drastically at the end because you are trying to maintain your average pace. If you focus on running your current racing tempo, the pace will always feel relaxed at the start of every interval.

The interval distance should be long enough that you feel some race-specific discomfort by the time you finish. The later you are in a workout, the sooner you'll experience this discomfort and the sooner you'll have to press in order to maintain the pace. But you shouldn't be dying during the last endurance interval. Rather, you should feel ready after a break of several minutes to run the speed intervals.

The endurance-speed workout is a prelude to the endurance workout. The endurance workout is specific to the later stages of a 5K or 10K race, because the pace-specific intervals are longer than they were in the endurance-speed

ENDURANCE-SPEED WORKOUT

1. Warm up for 15 minutes at mild-to-light exertion.

2. Run a set of pace-specific endurance intervals on the track (3 minutes for 5K or 5 minutes for 10K). Don't exceed the following heart rate limits for a 10K: elite runners 83 percent of maximum, competitive runners 82 percent, and recreational runners 81 percent. Don't exceed the following heart rate limits for a 5K: elite runners 85 percent of maximum, competitive runners 84 percent, and recreational runners 83 percent. Run the following number of intervals for a hard workout: high capacity 5, medium 5, and low 4. Run the following number of intervals for a moderate workout: high capacity 4, medium 4, and low 3. During the first three weeks, build the duration of the endurance interval by 30 seconds per week and reach the scheduled level on the third week. The intervals should be long enough to cause race-specific breathing by the third or fourth interval. Start each interval at a relaxed level. Adjust the interval distance to make your breathing during the last third of an interval specific to the second half of your race. Rest-jog for 80 to 90 seconds between intervals.

3. Run a set of pace-specific speed intervals (45 seconds for 5K or 90 seconds for 10K). Don't exceed the following heart rate limits for a 10K: elite runners 83 percent of maximum, competitive runners 82 percent, and recreational runners 81 percent. Don't exceed the following heart rate limits for a 5K: elite runners 85 percent of maximum, competitive runners 84 percent, and recreational runners 83 percent. Run the following number of intervals for a hard workout: high capacity 5, medium 5, and low 4. Run the following number of intervals for a moderate workout: high capacity 4, medium 4, and low 3.

4. Cool down at light-to-mild exertion for 5 minutes.

This is a tough workout to do because exertion climbs to race-specific intensity, which could be uncomfortable. It's important to realize, however, that these are not all-out intervals. Your exertion has to be meted out in precise dosages.

ENDURANCE WORKOUT

1. Warm up for 15 minutes at mild-to-light exertion.
2. Run a set of three pace-specific repetitions on the track or road (4 minutes for 5K or 8 minutes for 10K. Take a 3-minute rest jog between repetitions. Adjust the distance of the intervals to make your breathing during the last third of the interval specific to the second half of your race. The intervals should be long enough to cause race-specific breathing, depending on how hard you intend to run the second half of your goal-race. Think in terms of whether your breathing will be inaudible throughout, inaudible-to-heavy, or heavy-to-labored. Build exertion slowly after each rest interval, starting relaxed and increasing slowly to a race-specific breathing level. The overall workout effort could be moderate with two repetitions or hard with three repetitions.
3. Cool down for 15 minutes at light-to-mild exertion.

A sure way to tell if you are running too fast during an endurance workout is to track your times for the three repetitions. The first should be the slowest, the second should be significantly faster (because you have warmed up with the first rep), and the third should be the same pace as the second or a little faster. If you slow down on the last repetition, even though it feels about the same as the second repetition, then you went out too fast on the first or second repetition.

workout. Longer intervals at the same tempo are more intense. In this sense, the endurance workout is like a practice race because you have to hold the tempo without a break for a relatively long time.

You shouldn't run a hard endurance workout within the last two weeks before a goal-race. Even prior to the last two weeks, you should have decreased the number of endurance repetitions until you are running not more than one rep 10 days before your goal-race, with not more than three speed-specific intervals.

Taking the Next Step

Some years ago I had a conversation with one of my coaching peers. He had recently taken a new position coaching track at a local high school and he wanted me to explain how to set up endurance workouts for his milers. Ron knew how to run endurance workouts for the marathon, but he wasn't sure how to apply the endurance concept to a much shorter distance. Once I explained how to compress endurance intervals to fit the specific exertion structure of the mile, he got the idea and never needed my advice again. Moreover, his athletes began to perform at the statewide level because they had developed a fuller complement of racing abilities.

In your own training, you should now have an understanding of how to structure workouts to build ability for a goal-race. In the next chapter, I will step back again and consider the process of stringing workouts together to form a program. You will learn how to tailor a program to fit your particular needs, timeframe, and ability so you are well-prepared on race day.

CHAPTER 8

Tailoring 5K and 10K Programs

The days of one-size-fits-all training programs are over. They may have worked for some people in the past, but they often resulted in disaster for athletes who fell outside of their ability niche. To some extent, this could be true of the sample training programs in this chapter. They are designed for the recreational, competitive, and elite runners of varying fitness levels and backgrounds.

I realize that you may not fit this profile, either in terms of experience, ability, or goals. Thus, the program tables presented in this chapter are like the workout descriptions I presented in chapter 7. I only intend to show you possibilities for setting up a program. Once you understand the principles that underpin those possibilities, you should be able to tailor your own workouts and programs to fit your needs, goals, and training time frame.

Yearlong Training Programs

The programmatic process presupposes a minimal time frame for success. You can't expect your body to make the necessary succession of adaptations overnight. This is why I generally think of a training program as taking about a year to complete. As you'll see later in this chapter, shorter programs are definitely possible as long as you are willing to cut some corners.

For the moment, however, I would like to present some ideas related to progressive training within a yearlong time frame. A year is long enough to train incrementally, without radical increases in exertion. A program that you repeat on a yearly basis can give you a sense of stability, continuity, and progressive development as the same races and workouts come around again and again.

Workout Progressions

A yearlong training program can be a complex entity. In essence, a program is comprised of several workout progressions originating with individual base workouts. These separate progressions evolve from period to period, building a succession of abilities that culminate with peak ability in a goal-race.

Suppose you want to build your 10K tempo ability with a training progression. You could start your program with a workout that includes a number of pace-specific tempo intervals. If you're careful, you will derive adaptive value from the workout, as you would from any other. But because the workout is already pace-specific, it doesn't necessarily lend itself to significant adaptive progress. Of course, you could prolong the ability-building process by making the intervals longer and more intense, and by adding speed work to the mix. But eventually your body will become fully able to do the progression and, after that, you would have to begin again with a base workout.

As an alternative to beginning with pace-specific tempo training, you could begin with a much longer, slower workout designed to build your stamina. It would take time to introduce, establish, and adapt to this workout, but then you could introduce, establish, and adapt to a somewhat shorter and faster workout. By this method, it could take months before you come around to building pace-specific tempo for your 10K (see figure 8.1).

The main advantage to beginning a program with long, slow workouts is the way they increase your performance capacity during the process of base building, sharpening, and peaking. By the end of a program, you'll not only be able to run longer, tougher, pace-specific workouts but also faster races than you would have by beginning with pace-specific training instead of long, slow distance. This improved performance capacity develops out of the process of periodic training.

Periodicity leads eventually to a super-abundance of running energy. The process begins with workouts that force your body to adjust to increases in workout duration. As you run increasingly longer workouts, you maintain your effort relative to the limits of your expanding capacity. You don't exhaust yourself, but neither do you have much extra energy. Similarly, the goal of the sharpening period is to find a balance between shorter duration and higher exertion so you build new abilities without injury, illness, or exhaustion. Your training still demands lots of energy. But you are progressively building the capacity to run faster, despite a heavy training load.

After the heavy training of the base-building and sharpening periods, the program finally lightens up during the peaking period. Peaking allows your energy to soar as you radically shorten your workouts, reduce their overall effort, and decrease workout frequency. With the focus on peaking for 5K or 10K racing,

Pace exertion scale

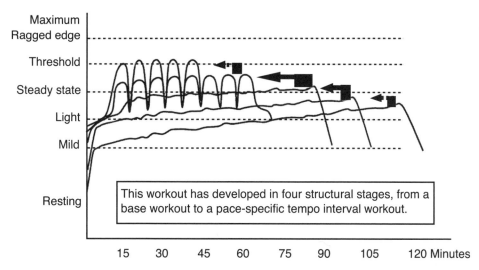

This workout has developed in four structural stages, from a base workout to a pace-specific tempo interval workout.

Figure 8.1 Given an initial base workout at the mild-to-light exertion level, this workout develops in stages (as indicated by the arrows), from a light exertion long run to a race-specific interval workout at the audible breathing threshold. The runner may have taken eight months to accomplish this adaptive progression.

some workout exertion could be at the audible breathing level. But all your workouts are sufficiently short and infrequent so that you have abundant energy whenever you train.

This abundant energy is a result of your long and arduous training earlier in the program. You might have achieved this adaptive effect with shorter base-building and sharpening periods. But you can't expect the same results by starting with a peaking schedule and no prior base. Nor can you expect the same abundance of energy to materialize with a sharpening schedule that demands a constant output of hard workouts that consume most of your running energy.

Thus, if you want abundant energy for a goal-race, you must play the programmatic game. A program builds a base of stamina, sharpens pace-specific abilities, and peaks your racing capacity. Ultimately, you'll have an abundance of energy for your goal-race as long as you are willing to reduce your training so your body super-adapts to prior programmatic stressors.

Four Training Progressions

At the beginning of a program, you should have a plan for the way your various workouts will evolve. For instance, a single stamina run could evolve into a shorter, faster steady-state workout, which becomes a shorter faster pace-specific tempo workout, and ultimately a still shorter and faster combination tempo-speed workout. You might say the entire progression is a stamina-tempo-speed progression, but I usually call it tempo-speed according to its ultimate race-specific purpose.

In this sense, you could construct the following ability-building progressions during a yearlong program: tempo-speed, power-endurance, and stamina. In this program, they all begin with stamina workouts in various weekly time slots. But those workouts evolve during the program to build a succession of abilities according to plan.

> **Stamina.** The purpose of this progression is to build your ability to run long and slow. As you adapt to long, slow workouts, you increase their duration through the base-building and sharpening periods. As you enter the peaking period before a goal-race, however, you back off on the frequency and duration of these long runs and use the energy you've gained through adaptation for other efforts,

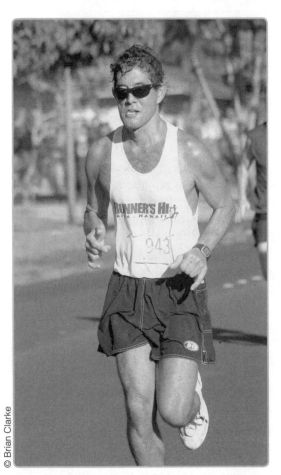

such as practice races and pace-specific endurance training. Though some of the workouts in your long-run time slot build endurance, you continue doing long runs on a less frequent basis throughout the program.

> **Recovery Run.** The recovery-run progression also builds stamina by virtue of the mild-to-light exertion nature of the workouts. Easy or moderate workouts are interspersed between major workouts, adding to your weekly mileage so you can approach the limits of your capacity for weekly running. Depending on your capacity and your ambition, you could do recovery runs as much as twice a day between your major workouts. You can also build other abilities besides stamina by adding hills and intervals to your recovery runs, provided these workouts are also easy enough to qualify as recovery runs.

> **Power-Endurance.** The power-endurance progression can begin with the same sort of workouts as a stamina progression, but you soon add hills to your long runs, which augments the muscle-strengthening process. As your power grows, the hill work takes on an intervallic nature, and your hill-running

A yearlong training program gives you enough time during a progression of training periods to build a full complement of racing abilities.

motion gradually becomes more vigorous. Eventually, you will combine tempo intervals on the flat with intervals in the hills, as you begin a process of phasing resistance training out and tempo training in. Ultimately, power workouts become endurance workouts as your tempo training is extended for progressively longer intervals, thereby simulating the specific discomfort of your goal-race.

> **Tempo-Speed.** The tempo-speed progression can also begin with long, slow, stamina training. But once you adapt to the duration of light-exertion running, you shorten the duration of the initial workout while raising your exertion. Depending on the time you have to train, you could restructure this workout several times, aiming at exertion that's specific to the tempo of your goal-race. You maintain a high-volume tempo regimen until the peaking period, when you markedly decrease the volume of tempo running while adding a little speed-specific training to the mix of tempo intervals.

I've chosen four separate progressions that combine a variety of ability-building purposes. They all begin by building stamina, so the workouts are somewhat indistinguishable initially. Once you begin changing workout purpose, their exertion structure also changes according to the abilities you intend to build. There is nothing magic about the way the progressions develop. I could have made an endurance workout out of a tempo workout, for instance, instead of making an endurance workout out of a hill workout.

The previous chapter described a number of workouts that could fit within these training progressions. Those workout descriptions are a lot like recipes you might use to prepare a meal. In this sense, a training program is a complex recipe for a series of meals. How will the exertion structure of the base workouts change from one training period to another? What abilities will you build, assuming the ultimate purpose of the program will be to build a full complement of pace-specific abilities for your goal-race?

Once you have a handle on how to structure various ability-building workouts, there is no reason why you shouldn't create your own progressions that fulfill your own logic and training rationale. Similarly, you may have a set of favorite workouts that will substitute for mine. As long as you can see the logic of doing your workouts, and as long as they work as ability-building substitutes, I encourage you to do your own familiar workouts.

Short-Term Training Programs

I personally prefer developing and running yearlong training programs. I like tweaking them from year to year, always aiming at running an ideal program and an ideal goal-race. I realize, however, that you may not want to invest a year to prepare for a single goal-race. You may want to train for a race that's coming up in, say, 12 weeks. How can you compress a year of training into a short-term program? The answer is, you can't; at least not without cutting corners. Many of my athletes join one of my three-month training programs with little or no background, and they often stop training after running their goal-race. Such short-term, ad hoc training programs can't be as effective as a series of yearlong programs that develop performance capacity progressively from year to year. It takes years to reach one's full racing potential. Nonetheless, if you only have 12 weeks to train for a race, it is possible to create a short-term program to fit your training time frame.

A short-term program should take advantage of your recent training background by building new abilities on the ones you've recently built. Unless you are starting from scratch, you'll have at least a minimal background of training upon which you can build a program. This background constitutes your training profile.

I will assist you in assessing your personal ability profile later in this chapter. I will also assist you in constructing a tailored program that suits your needs, goals, and time frame. Meanwhile, the following sample programs will show you how to construct a short-term training program based on an ability profile.

Training and Racing Profiles

If you are an elite runner, you've been training and racing for awhile. That background has given you a repertoire of racing abilities, which are part of your runner profile. Your profile gives you a starting point for deciding which workouts you should do as a next step toward becoming a more effective racer. Unless you've covered all the bases with your recent training, there are abilities you could still build with your next training program.

I will lead you through a process of setting up the workouts to build these abilities at the end of this chapter. Here, I want to develop the profile idea with three examples. In each case, I've included a short-term training program that meets a specific ability profile, including:

> A recreational runner in fair condition who has a 10K goal-race in 10 weeks and aims to finish under 60 minutes (Runner A).

> A competitive runner with an extensive background of long and slow running who has a 10K goal-race in 14 weeks and aims to finish in less than 38 minutes (Runner B).

> An elite runner with extensive experience but little recent training who is making a comeback and has a 5K goal-race in 20 weeks (Runner C).

Each training program should be understood in context with these basic profiles. Thus, their applicability to your particular circumstances will depend on how well you match the profile. A program description is included as part of the profile, and it should be studied in conjunction with the workout summary table that accompanies it.

RUNNER A

Profile
Female athlete in fair shape who has never trained competitively. Her training has consisted of sporadic easy to moderate training during the past year.

Race
10K Run for Cancer

Time line
10 weeks

Goals
To improve her training and racing competency; to lower her 10K time from 65 minutes to less than 60 minutes; to enjoy the training; and to survive without getting injured.

Current abilities
Some stamina

Abilities to develop:
Continue working on stamina while developing tempo and power at the steady-state level

Training schedule (60-48-60-hour schedule)
Tuesday-Thursday-Sunday (moderate to hard workouts)

Monday-Wednesday-Friday (easy runs)

Saturday (day off)

Training regimen
> 15-minute jogging warm-up at the start of all workouts

> Three moderate to hard workouts per week, focusing on the following:

1. Steady-state tempo interval workout. (She will run a variety of short interval distances at a quick, relaxed tempo as a step up from her usual slow training pace.)

2. Combination hill and interval workout. (This workout will begin with some steady-state intervals on a track. She will introduce hill training at her slowest jogging pace initially. If she feels strong enough later in the program, she may use a slow bouncing motion at her steady-state level.)

(continued)

3. Long run (She will run this workout at the conversational level, increasing workout duration from 50 to 90 minutes during the first four weeks of the program.)

4. Practice races (She will run a series of practice races during the program, focusing on developing her racing skills.)

Runner A is a recreational runner with 10 weeks to train for a 10K goal-race. This athlete has never trained competitively, but she is in fair shape at the start of the program. Lacking the discipline to train by herself, she has the commitment of a friend to support her in doing the training together.

These buddies have been training sporadically for a year with easy to moderate workouts and occasional fun run races. They have never done hard workouts, but they aim to run their 10K goal-race together as a hard effort with the goal of improving their best 10K time. They believe their previous best 10K is in the 65-minute range, and they want to run a sub-60-minute 10K.

The 10-week program is designed to increase their training and racing competency. They will build the duration of their long runs, hills, and intervals, and they will participate in several practice races. Since they are used to running mostly easy workouts, the program will challenge them to build a long-run base while incorporating hills and intervals to prepare for a sub-60-minute 10K on a moderately hilly course.

In order to do this program, they have each purchased a basic POLAR heart rate monitor. They have measured distances of 50, 100, 200, 300, and 800 meters in a grassy city park. They know their maximum heart rate from having done the max test described in chapter 1. They have agreed with one another to stay at least five beats per minute below their audible breathing level during their hills and intervals. Otherwise, they will simply focus on a quick, relaxed pace during tempo intervals.

They have agreed to meet for their hill training at a location that happens to be within a five-minute jog of a high school track. The basic hill workout calls for them to do a 15-minute warm-up, some quick and relaxed tempo intervals on the track, and then a loosely structured meandering run in the surrounding hills. There are some trails in the area, and they are encouraged to run them. They may exceed the recommended time in the hills only if they are able to recover in time for their interval workout 48 hours later.

They have read this book and answered the assessment questions related to scheduling and capacity. They will do a 60-48-60-hour schedule of three moderate workouts a week, which is in line with their medium capacity for exertion. This buddy couple has agreed to run three off-day, easy workouts on the weeknights between their major weekly workouts on Tuesday and Thursday evenings and Sunday morning. Since they work in the same building, they plan to start and finish the recovery runs from their workplace immediately after work. The off-day recovery run will consist of a slow 35-minute jog on the same course they have been running together for some time.

They are scheduled to do a fun run 5K at the end of the first week of training. They aren't in shape for a best effort in the race, but it offers them an opportunity to practice aspects of the race they want to do at the end of the program, including visualizing the racecourse by running it slowly the week before, adopting a conscious routine of proper rest and nutrition the last few days before the race, as well as a proper warm-up the morning of the race and a slow cool-down afterwards. They can use their pace for the race as an indication of their current pace for their intervals. And they can practice taking care of themselves after the race by changing to warm, dry clothes and by drinking sufficient liquids to be quickly and adequately rehydrated.

Because they have no experience with interval training, they are scheduled to practice a quick and relaxed, steady-state tempo as a step up from their usual slow training pace. Quick and relaxed also happens to be the tempo of their 10K goal-race. The first interval workouts in the program are designed to introduce intervals to them so they can practice the rhythm of tempo intervals and rest intervals without stopping or walking. They need to learn the right tempo and allow their bodies to get used to the new interval exertion structure.

Because they are also inexperienced with hill training, they have been advised to begin with simply getting up the hills at their slowest pace. If they feel strong enough later in the program, they may increase their exertion to the slow-bouncing-motion level. The first workouts in this progression are designed to introduce them to running uphill. At the introductory week-1 level, they will alternate jogging with walking. Each will jog at the other's walking pace so they both learn to hold an appropriately slow jogging pace in the hills.

The long-run progression will be most familiar to them in terms of its exertion pattern, which is simply slow and conversational. They will start the long run from various locations, which they have scheduled to fit the duration of the program. Some long runs will have hills to complement their hill training, and some will be on trails for variety. The most challenging aspect of the long-run progression will be the growing duration of the workouts, from their current longest of 50 minutes to 90 minutes.

Table 8.1 follows the progression of major Tuesday, Thursday, and Sunday workouts during the 10-week training. Easy workouts are not shown here, but they are run on Monday, Wednesday, and Friday afternoons. There is no workout on Saturday.

TABLE 8.1   10-Week 10K Program for Recreational Runners

Week	Tuesday (Hills)	Thursday (Intervals)	Sunday (Long Runs)
1	Warm up 15 min very slow Jog slowly up a gradual, 150m hill four times, jogging slowly down Run a long uphill, alternating 2 min walking and 2 min jogging for 16 min	Practice the same warm-up as Sunday's race, employing a very slow pace in the same warm-up area Jog the 5K racecourse, visualizing how to run it, given its layout and features Plan how to take care of yourself before, during, and after the race	**5K Practice Race** Warm up at very slow pace for 25 min Run 5K as a test effort. Run slow enough that breathing remains inaudible Cool down for 10 min and take care of yourself as planned
2	Warm up 15 min very slow. On track or measured course, alternate 4 × 100 at quick, relaxed pace with 100 m very slow Jog hilly course alternating 3-min jog and walk for 20 min	Warm up 15 min very slow Run the following tempo intervals at quick, relaxed pace, and the rest jog very slow without stopping: 10 × 50; with 25m rest 6 × 100; jog 50 sec 4 × 200; jog 50 sec 10 min cool-down	70 min run at mild-to-light exertion Include one long hill at light exertion
3	Warm up 15 min very slow On track or measured course, 6 × 100 at quick, relaxed pace, 75% of maximum Jog hilly course 45 min	Warm up 15 min very slow Quick, relaxed tempo intervals: 4 × 100; jog 50 sec 4 × 200; jog 50 sec 4 × 300; jog 60 sec 10 min slow cool-down	80 min run at mild-to-light exertion Include 20 min of uphill jogging at light exertion
4	Warm up 15 min very slow On track or measured course, 8 × 100 at quick, relaxed pace, 75% of maximum Jog hilly course 50 min	Warm up 15 min very slow Quick, relaxed tempo intervals: 4 × 200; jog 50 sec 8 × 300; jog 60 sec 10 min slow cool-down	90 min run at mild-to-light exertion Include 25 min of uphill jogging at light exertion
5	Warm up 15 min very slow On track or measured course, 8 × 100 at quick, relaxed pace, 75% of maximum Jog hilly course 30 min	Practice warming up in same warm-up area as Sunday's race Jog key parts of the 8K racecourse, visualizing exertion levels Plan how to take care of yourself before, during, and after the race	**8K Practice Race** Warm up at very slow pace for 20 min. Add 3 × 50 m at quick, relaxed pace Focus on quick, relaxed start; don't hear breathing before halfway; finish with audible breathing, feeling strong Cool down for 15 min and take care of yourself as planned
6	Warm up 15 min very slow On track or measured course, 8 × 50 at quick, relaxed pace, 75% of maximum Jog 10 min	Warm up 15 min very slow Quick, relaxed tempo intervals: 10 × 200; jog 60 sec 10 min slow cool-down	90 min run at mild-to-light exertion Include 20 min of uphill jogging at light exertion

Week	Tuesday (Hills)	Thursday (Intervals)	Sunday (Long Runs)

7	Warm up 15 min very slow
	
	On track or measured course, 6 × 200 at quick, relaxed pace, 75% of maximum
	
	Jog hilly course 60 min
		Warm up 15 min very slow
		
		Quick, relaxed tempo intervals:
		
		  4 × 300; jog 60 sec
		
		  1 × 800; jog 3 min
		
		  3 × 200 at rapid, pressed pace; jog 60 sec
		
		10 min slow cool-down
			90 min run at mild-to-light exertion
			
			Include 30 min of uphill jogging at light exertion

8	Warm up 15 min very slow On track or measured course, 8 × 100 at quick, relaxed pace, 75% of maximum Jog hilly course 30 min	Practice warming up at same warm-up area as Sunday's race Jog the racecourse, visualizing exertion levels and timing points Plan how to take care of yourself before, during, and after the race	**5K Practice Race** Warm up at very slow pace for 20 min. Add 3 × 50 at quick, relaxed pace. Run first mile at 10K pace; run last two miles at audible breathing level; finish feeling strong Cool down for 20 min and practice taking care of yourself after the race

9	Warm up 15 min very slow
	
	On track or measured course, 6 × 100 at quick, relaxed pace (75% of maximum) and 4 × 100 at rapid, pressed pace (80% of maximum)
	
	Jog 10 min
		Warm up 15 min very slow
		
		Quick, relaxed tempo intervals:
		
		  2 × 300; jog 60 sec
		
		  1 × 800; jog 3 min
		
		  2 × 200 at rapid, pressed pace; jog 60 sec
		
		5 min slow cool-down
			75 min visualization run on goal-race course at mild-to-light exertion. See the course as you will run it from the warm-up to the cool-down.

10	Warm up 15 min very slow On track or measured course, 6 × 100 at quick, relaxed pace (75% of maximum) and 4 × 100 at rapid, pressed pace (80% of maximum) Jog 10 min	Warm up 15 min very slow Quick, relaxed tempo intervals: 4 × 300; jog 60 sec 5 min slow cool-down	**10K Goal-Race** Feel eager to race, light and fit Warm up as before and start at quick, relaxed pace Run the uphills slower than the down, maintaining the same gradually increasing heart rate throughout, with audible breathing after the midpoint only Finish feeling strong Cool down for 10 min and take care of yourself as usual

RUNNER B

Profile

A competitive female runner who has developed a broad base of stamina during the past five years. She runs 55 to 70 miles per week, often including double workouts. She usually gives herself an easy day before a race or a long run of 12 to 16 miles, but she feels lazy for her other workouts, managing to run only 6 to 8 miles before running out of energy. Runner B races once or twice a month, but she is frustrated with her times in the 40-minute range for 10K.

Race

10K Heart Run

Time line

14 weeks

Goal

To reestablish her ability to run a 10K race in 38 minutes

Current abilities

Mostly stamina, with some endurance from frequent racing

Abilities to develop

Power, tempo, speed, and endurance

New training schedule

Tuesday-Thursday-Sunday (hard workouts)

Monday-Wednesday-Friday-Saturday (a single 40- to 50-minute easy workout)

New training regimen

> 15-minute warm-up at mild-to-light exertion before all workouts (25- to 30-minute warm-up before all races), including three or four light-exertion, 50-meter pickups at a pace between her warm-up pace and training or racing pace.

> Three hard workouts on the 48-48-72-hour schedule.

   1. Endurance workout (On Sundays she will do a long run for stamina, alternating with a race, or a sustained tempo workout on the actual racecourse. The races and the sustained tempo workout at her audible breathing threshold will build endurance.)

   2. Tempo workout (On Thursdays she will do a high-volume tempo interval workout, building to 24 × 400 meters by the sixth week. Then the

number of intervals becomes increasingly fewer and sharper, leading up to the goal-race. There is a strict heart rate limit to all these intervals.)

3. Power-speed workout (This is a combination hill and track workout. Some hills will be long and slow; others will be short and more vigorous. The intervals on the track will be short and up-tempo, but not so fast that she will finish feeling winded.)

Runner B is a competitive runner who has a 10K goal-race in 14 weeks. This female athlete is in good shape from having built a broad base of long, slow running during the past several years. She races at least once or twice a month, but she is frustrated with times in the 40-minute range for 10K, believing she can still run at least 38:00. She is used to high mileage, hard workouts, and very hard races.

The answers to this runner's personal assessment indicate that she has a tremendous base of long, slow running, with very little recent pace-specific training for the 10K. She considers her frequent racing as her "speed work," but her times have leveled off at about 40 minutes, which is slower than her best of 36 minutes seven years ago. She believes that her age has slowed her down (she is in her early 40s). But she also thinks she can still run faster than 40 minutes for 10K.

Because she loves running, she does a lot of it. She runs every day and often twice a day. She rarely runs less than 50 miles a week—even when she races—and she is often in the 60- to 70-mile range. As a result, she usually feels lazy for her workouts, managing to run only between 6 and 8 miles before she runs out of energy. Sometimes she gives herself a couple of easy days before a race or a longer run of 12 to 16 miles. She considers herself to be primarily a marathoner, but she yearns for a return to the days when she was competitive at the 10K, too.

Her 14-week program leading up to a 10K goal-race will be a radical departure from recent training. It will have distinct hard and easy workouts. Her main challenge initially will be to give up some of her weekly mileage in favor of a shorter hard–easy regimen. She is willing to run hard workouts, but she will resist cutting back to a single slow-and-easy 40-minute workout in between hard workouts. Unless she can discipline herself to feel ready for her hard workouts, however, her 48-48-72-hour hard workout schedule will not work, and the program will devolve into an ineffective parody of her recent long-slow training.

Since she has a well-developed mileage base and a dearth of recent pace-specific training, the program will focus on race-specificity from the outset. The endurance workout on Sundays is run on the same moderately hilly

(continued)

10K course of her goal-race. The first mile is a continuation of a 15-minute warm-up. The second and third miles are a little quicker, but still only at low-level steady state. The last 5K is timed and held as close as possible to an 80 percent heart rate limit. The goal during this workout is to build exertion without getting into audible breathing. This is not an endurance workout per se, but an opportunity to practice holding exertion as close as possible to the audible breathing level, without exceeding it. She is advised to start at a different mile-mark of the course each week so she learns how to run the entire course at 10K tempo.

The athlete has a sophisticated heart rate monitor with a computer interface. She can use it to compare key workouts, such as the sustained 5K runs. She should establish a target heart rate and a maximum limit for the workout after the first couple of weeks. Times for the workout should gradually fall during the training period at the same average heart rate. In fact, one heart rate graph should be identical to any of the others in the series. Thus, the monitor will provide a way of measuring adaptive progress as well as keeping her at the proper target during the workouts.

The tempo intervals on Thursday morning will increase in number until she is running 24 quarters (approximate 10K) at tempo by the sixth week. There-after, tempo interval workouts will become increasingly shorter and sharper, leading up to the goal-race. The key to running this workout is to be very clear and disciplined about the heart rate limit for each workout. It's tempting to run faster than the limit, because the limit is well within her capacity. A faster pace, however, isn't necessarily a more adaptive pace. All she needs is to see improvement (faster times) at the target heart rate, because improvement in the workouts means improvement in the races.

Because she has run mostly on level ground lately, she has comparatively little muscle strength. Her third workout progression, therefore, will be a hill regimen on a circuit course that will help her regulate the number and variety of hill intervals. She will start with slow and gentle hills and gradually build to a bouncing motion at a steady-state level. Some hills will be long enough to force a slow pace; other hills will be short enough for a more vigorous bounc-ing motion. She understands that her hills and intervals could be injurious, and that she doesn't have time to waste with injury layoffs before her race in 14 weeks. See table 8.2 for a sample 14-week 10K program for a competi-tive runner.

The schedule calls for her to run hard workouts three days a week in the morning. She will do only one easy workout of 40 to 50 minutes on all the other days. She must run slowly enough on the easy days that she is ready for her hard workouts, with enough energy to complete them without undo fatigue.

She will use her heart rate monitor to establish and abide by target ranges for all of her hard and easy workouts.

The assumption is that a runner at this level knows how to warm up and cool down. She should run a 15-minute mild-to-light exertion warm-up before all intervals and a 25- to 30-minute warm-up before all races. Every warm-up should include three or four light-exertion, 50-meter pickups at a pace that builds from her warm-up pace to her training or racing pace.

TABLE 8.2   14-Week 10K Program for Competitive Runners With Extensive Basic Background

Week	Tuesday morning (Power-Speed)	Thursday morning (Tempo-Speed)	Sunday morning (long run, race, or endurance)
1	6 × 200 at 75% 30 min hill circuit 3 × 100 at 75%	14 × 400 at 75-77% Rest for 60 sec at a very slow jog Cool down 10 min	10K run on goal-race course, with second 5K at 77-79% and no audible breathing
2	8 × 200 at 75% 40 min hill circuit 3 × 100 at 75%	18 × 400 at 75-77% Rest for 60 sec at a very slow jog. Cool down 10 min	Long run, 16 miles at 55-65%
3	6 × 300 at 75% 50 min hill circuit 3 × 100 at 75%	20 × 400 at 75-77% Rest for 60 sec at a very slow jog Cool down 10 min	10K run on goal-race course, with second 5K at 77-79% and no audible breathing
4	8 × 3 00 at 75% 60 min hill circuit 4 × 100 at 75%	22 × 400 at 75-77% Rest for 60 sec at a very slow jog Cool down 10 min	Long run, 18 miles at 55-65%
5	8 × 300 at 75% 60 min hill circuit 4 × 100 at 75%	24 × 400 at 75-77% Rest for 60 sec at a very slow jog Cool down 10 min	10K run on goal-race course, with second 5K at 77-79% and no audible breathing
6	4 × 300 at 75% 20 min hill circuit 2 × 100 at 75%	**Visualization Run on 8K course** See the race as you want to run it, regarding the features of the course and your exertion at various points	**Practice 8K Race** Run the race exactly as you envisioned it, and feel great about the experience
7	60 min recovery run	6 × 800 at 76-78% Rest for 75 sec at a very slow jog Cool down 10 min	Long run, 16 miles at 55-65%
8	8 × 300 at 75% 40 min hill circuit 4 × 100 at 75%	5 × 1,200 at 78-80% Rest for 90 sec at a very slow jog Cool down 10 min	10K run on goal-race course, with second 5K at 77-79% and no audible breathing

(continued)

129

TABLE 8.2 *(continued)*

Week	Tuesday morning (Power-Speed)	Thursday morning (Tempo-Speed)	Sunday morning (long run, race, or endurance)
9	8 × 300 at 75% 40 min hill circuit 4 × 100 at 75%	5 × 1,200 at 78-80% Rest for 90 sec at a very slow jog Cool down 10 min	Long run, 18 miles at 55-65%
10	**Visualization Run** 4 × 100 at 75%	**Visualization Run on 5K course** See the race as you want to run it, regarding the features of the course and your exertion at various points	**Practice 5K Race** Run the race exactly as you envisioned it, and feel great about the experience
11	Recovery run of 50 min	4 × 1,200 at 80-82% Rest for 90 sec at a very slow jog Cool down 10 min	Long run, 16 miles at 55-65%
12	12 × 400 at 79-81% Rest for 60 sec at a very slow jog Cool down 10 min	3 × 1,200 at 80-82% Rest for 90 sec at a very slow jog Cool down 10 min	10K run on goal-race course, with second 5K at 77-79% and no audible breathing
13	8 × 400 at 79-81% Rest for 60 sec at a very slow jog Cool down 10 min	8 × 100 at rapid, pressed tempo Rest for 60 seconds at a very slow jog Cool down 10 min	Moderate run, 8 miles at 55-65%
14	60 min taper jog	40 min taper jog	**10K Goal-Race** Run the race exactly as you have envisioned it during your sustained 5K efforts, and feel great about the experience

RUNNER C

Profile
Elite runner who is making a comeback after a six-year hiatus in which weekly training consisted mostly of three or four easy workouts. He is eight pounds over optimal racing weight.

Race
5K Marshall County Fun Run

Time line
20 weeks

Goal
To run a 5K in 17 minutes or less as soon as possible

Current abilities
Some stamina. He is untrained but has outstanding natural talent.

Abilities to develop
Continue working on stamina, develop power, tempo, speed, and endurance

Scheduling progression
Weeks 1 to 4 (84-84-hour schedule)
> Wednesday-Sunday (hard workouts)
> Monday-Tuesday-Thursday-Friday-Saturday (30-minute easy run)

Weeks 5 to 14 (60-48-60-hour workout schedule)
> Tuesday-Thursday-Sunday (hard workouts)
> Monday-Wednesday-Friday-Saturday (30- to 45-minute easy run)

Weeks 15 to 20
> Sunday (hard workout)
> Tuesday-Thursday (moderate workouts)
> Monday-Wednesday-Friday-Saturday (45-minute easy runs)

Training regimen
> 15-minute warm-up at mild-to-light exertion before all training (25- to 30-minute warm-up before all races), including three or four light-exertion, 50-meter pickups at a pace between warm-up pace and training or racing pace.
> Weeks 1 to 4:
   1. Long run (at mild-to-light exertion, starting at 60 minutes and building to 90).

(continued)

2. Tempo interval workout (at a quick and relaxed steady-state level, starting with 800s and building to 1,200s).

> Weeks 5 to 14:

1. Long run (building duration from 100 minutes to two hours on Sundays when he doesn't run a practice race or test effort).
2. Tempo interval workout (dropping from 8 to 5 × 1,200s at 79 percent of maximum, including 3 × 200 at 79 percent).
3. Power–speed workout (on the track and in the hills, with short speed intervals before and after a 20- to 60-minute hill circuit run).

He may postpone the hill workout several weeks until he can begin without major risk of overtraining.

> Weeks 15 to 20:

1. Long run (decreases to 90 minutes the week before the goal race).
2. Tempo interval workout (dropping the number of 1,200s to one at 84 percent of maximum, plus 3 × 200 at 84 percent of maximum, the week before the race).
3. Power-speed workout (the hill circuit is replaced by 800-meter track intervals during the 14th week).

Runner C refrains from racing during the first eight weeks so that he can establish a base of long workouts and return to racing weight. He should not add hills after week five unless he has survived to that point without injury or illness. After the first eight weeks, the program continues by alternating a race or a test effort with a staple long run on Sunday mornings.

This athlete is in a rush to get in shape and relive past glories. He doesn't realize how much he's lost during his racing and training hiatus. He's eight pounds over his former racing weight, and it will take time to lose that weight while maintaining his energy for training. Moreover, it will take time to reestablish the training base he once had. His biggest challenge will be to ease into his training over a period of several months, being satisfied with his performance in early races without expecting to peak for them.

His program calls for three distinct training periods of eight weeks, five weeks, and five weeks, each of which leads up to a race, culminating with the 5K goal-race. He will run two hard workouts a week, initially: a long run and a steady-state interval workout. He can shift to three hard workouts a week after the first four weeks, provided he has lost four pounds by then and he survives without illness or injury. He will hold a 60-48-60-hour hard workout schedule until the last five weeks, when he will gradually back off to two moderate workouts and a hard workout as he approaches his 5K goal-race.

With 20 weeks to train, he has time to settle gradually into a training regimen. He should refrain from racing during the first eight-week training period while he works to establish a base of long workouts. By then he should be back to racing weight and ready to test himself in a race, relying on his base and his natural talent. After the first eight weeks, the program continues with two-week couplets, alternating a race or a test-effort with a staple long run on Sunday mornings. The test-efforts are mental toughening and pacing exercises. They should be run with a heart rate monitor in hand and a clear idea of the various upper limits for each segment of the test effort. Depending on his energy after a race or test effort, he can run an additional 20 to 40 minutes at a slow pace.

The initial tempo workout progression (on Wednesday/Thursday) is an opportunity to build a base of steady-state tempo running. It starts with six quick, relaxed 800s and builds progressively to eight 1,200s by the sixth week. After the first practice race, the number of 1200s drops back to six and the intensity increases to 79% of maximum—as quick as possible without audible breathing. The last part of this new workout is a set of three 200s at the same 79% of maximum. As the number of 1,200s drops from six to five to four, the heart rate limit rises to a high of 84% of maximum, which should simulate the breathing and intensity of the second mile of a 5K.

The power-speed progression begins on Tuesdays after the fourth week, provided the athlete has lost four pounds and has not lost time to colds or injury. This progression can be postponed several weeks or more until the runner is in shape to begin without causing major overtraining difficulties. The power workout is a hill interval workout on a course that offers a variety of interesting hills of 50 to 300 meters. The shorter the hill the faster or more vigorous the running motion, without exceeding the inaudible breathing level. See table 8.3 for a sample 20-week 5K program for elite runners.

If this runner is thinking about winning his age division immediately, he is probably competing in a racing backwater. He must realize that, to have an impact in a truly competitive age division against other runners who have been training consistently for several years, he will have to take a long-term view to his training and racing. He should be patient with himself and work hard to expand his base during the next several years.

TABLE 8.3 20-Week 5K Program for Elite Runners With Little Recent Background

Week	Monday p.m.	Tuesday p.m.	Wednesday p.m.	Thursday p.m.	Friday p.m.	Saturday a.m.	Sunday a.m.
1	Easy run, 30 min	Easy run, 30 min	6 × 800 at 75% with rest jog of 80 sec	Easy run, 30 min	Easy run, 30 min	Easy run, 30 min	60 min at mild-to-light exertion
2	Easy run, 30 min	Easy run, 30 min	7 × 800 at 75% with rest jog of 80 sec	Easy run, 30 min	Easy run, 30 min	Easy run, 30 min	70 min at mild-to-light exertion
3	Easy run, 30 min	Easy run, 30 min	8 × 800 at 75% with rest jog of 80 sec	Easy run, 30 min	Easy run, 30 min	Easy run, 30 min	80 min at mild-to-light exertion
4	Easy run, 30 min	Easy run, 30 min	6 × 1200 at 75% with rest jog of 80 sec	Easy run, 30 min	Easy run, 30 min	Easy run, 30 min	90 min at mild-to-light exertion
5	Easy run, 30 min	6 × 200 at 75%; jog 200 40 min hill circuit with hills at 75% 4 × 100 at 75%	Easy run, 30 min	7 x 1200 at 75% with rest jog of 80 sec	Easy run, 30 min	Easy run, 30 min	100 min at mild-to-light exertion
6	Easy run, 30 min	6 × 200 at 75%; jog 200 30 min hill circuit with hills at 75% 4 × 100 at 75%	Easy run, 30 min	8 × 1200 at 75% with rest jog of 80 sec	Easy run, 30 min	Easy run, 30 min	110 min at mild-to-light exertion
7	Easy run, 30 min	6 × 200 at 75%; jog 200 40 min hill circuit with hills at 75% 4 × 100 at 75%	Easy run, 30 min	8 × 1200 at 75% with rest jog of 80 sec	Easy run, 30 min	Easy run, 30 min	120 min at mild-to-light exertion

Week	Monday p.m.	Tuesday p.m.	Wednesday p.m.	Thursday p.m.	Friday p.m.	Saturday a.m.	Sunday a.m.
8	Easy run, 30 min	6 × 200 at 75%; jog 200 20 min hill circuit with hills at 75% 4 × 100 at 75%	Easy run, 30 min	Moderate run, 60-70 min, including visualization of Sunday's 5K race-course	Easy run, 30 min	Easy run, 30 min	**5K Practice Race** Run the race exactly as you envisioned it, and feel great about the experience
9	Easy run, 40 min	3 × 200 at 70%; jog 200 30 min hill circuit with hills at 78% 2 × 100 at 78%	Easy run, 40 min	6 × 1,200 at 80%; jog 90 sec 3 × 200 at 80%; jog 60 sec	Easy run, 45 min	Easy run, 40 min	120 min at light exertion
10	Easy run, 40 min	6 × 200 at 77%; jog 200 60 min hill circuit with hills at 77% 4 × 100 at 77%	Easy run, 40 min	6 × 1,200 at 80%; jog 90 sec 3 × 200 at 80%; jog 60 sec	Easy run, 45 min	Easy run, 40 min	**5K Test Effort** Run first mile at 75%, second 1.5 miles at 80%, last mile at 85%
11	Easy run, 40 min	6 × 200 at 77%; jog 200 60 min hill circuit with hills at 77% 4 × 100 at 77%	Easy run, 40 min	6 × 1,200 at 80%; jog 90 sec 3 × 200 at 80%; jog 60 sec	Easy run, 45 min	Easy run, 40 min	120 min at light exertion
12	Easy run, 40 min	6 × 200 at 77%; jog 200 20 min hill circuit with hills at 77% 4 × 100 at 75%	Easy run, 40 min	Moderate run, 60-70 min	Easy run, 45 min	Easy run, 40 min	**8K Practice Race** Run the race exactly as you envisioned it, and feel great about the experience

(continued)

TABLE 8.3 *(continued)*

Week	Monday p.m.	Tuesday p.m.	Wednesday p.m.	Thursday p.m.	Friday p.m.	Saturday a.m.	Sunday a.m.
13	Easy run, 40 min	Moderate run, 60 min	Easy run, 40 min	5 × 1,200 at 82%; jog 90 sec 3 × 200 at 82%; jog 60 sec	Easy run, 45 min	Easy run, 40 min	120 min at light exertion
14	Easy run, 40 min	6 × 200 at 75%; jog 200 3 × 800 at 80% with 2 min jog 4 × 100 at 75%	Easy run, 40 min	5 × 1,200 at 82%; jog 90 sec 3 × 200 at 82%; jog 60 sec	Easy run, 45 min	Easy run, 40 min	**4-Mile Test Effort** Run first 2 miles at 75%, next 1.5 miles at 80%, last half mile at 88%
15	Easy run, 40 min	6 × 200 at 75%; jog 200 3 × 800 at 80% with 2 min jog 4 × 100 at 75%	Easy run, 40 min	5 × 1,200 at 84%; jog 90 sec 3 × 200 at 82%; jog 60 sec	Easy run, 45 min	Easy run, 40 min	120 min at light exertion
16	Easy run, 40 min	4 × 200 at 75%; jog 200 1 × 800 at 80% with 2 min jog 2 × 100 at 75%	Easy run, 40 min	Moderate run, 60-70 min	Easy run, 45 min	Easy run, 40 min	**5K Practice Race** Run the race exactly as you envisioned it, and feel great about the experience
17	Easy run, 40 min	Moderate run, 60 min	Easy run, 40 min	4 × 1,200 at 84%; jog 90 sec 3 × 200 at 84%; jog 60 sec	Easy run, 45 min	Easy run, 40 min	120 min at light exertion
18	Easy run, 40 min	4 × 200 at 75%; jog 200 3 × 800 at 83% with 2 min jog 2 × 100 at 75%	Easy run, 40 min	3 × 1,200 at 84%; jog 90 sec 3 × 200 at 84%; jog 60 sec	Easy run, 45 min	Easy run, 40 min	**2-Mile Test Effort** Run first mile at 80%, next mile at 88%

Week	Monday p.m.	Tuesday p.m.	Wednesday p.m.	Thursday p.m.	Friday p.m.	Saturday a.m.	Sunday a.m.
19	Easy run, 40 min	4 × 200 at 75%; jog 200 1 × 800 at 80% with 2 min jog 2 × 100 at 75%	Easy run, 40 min	1 × 1,200 at 84%; jog 90 sec 3 × 200 at 84%; jog 60 sec	Easy run, 45 min	Easy run, 40 min	90 min at light exertion
20	Easy run, 40 min	3 × 200 at 75%; jog 200 1 × 400 at 80% with 2 min jog 2 × 100 at 75%	Easy run, 40 min	Very easy run, 30 min	Very easy run, 20 min		**5K Goal Race** Run the race exactly as you envisioned it, and feel great about the experience

Tailoring a Program to Fit Your Racing Time Frame

Some athletes focus their training on a variety of races, changing their training according to the distance of their next race. If they are training for a long race like a marathon, for instance, they tend to train long, too. Athletes who vary their training according to a succession of random racing distances, can lose the benefit of a training program that builds progressively from training period to training period.

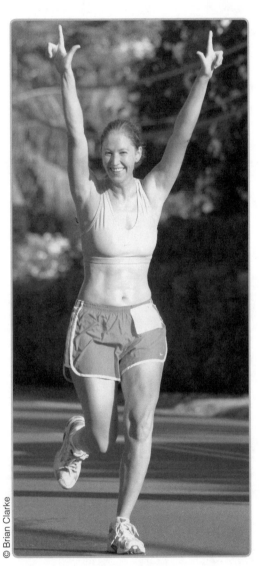

I recommend that you train for one goal-race during a training program, focusing your training progressively on that race. You can run other races during the program but, with the exception of tapering and recovering, you won't change your training for those races.

With these ideas in mind, your next step is to consider the races you would like to run during the next year. Table 8.4 will give you a way to visualize the distribution of those races.

Which race or races are most important to you? Please circle those races on table 8.4. Some athletes make few, if any, distinctions in the importance of their races. Either they consider them all very important or they consider few, if any, as important. If this applies to you, you have some choices to make if you are going to build a training program around a single goal-race.

Please circle the races on table 8.4 that you consider "goal-races" in the sense that your performance in them is very important or more important than the others. Are they clumped together or spread apart? Does their distribution suggest ways to build training programs leading up to them?

Beyond a consideration of your goal-race, you should also consider the frequency of your other races. How many races would you like to do during the year? Keep in mind you are creating a training program, not a racing program. If you intend to race every other week during the year, you are

A great race is one in which you raise your hands at the finish and exclaim, "Yes! *That was a great race.*" You know it because you've done exactly what you intended.

Table 8.4 Races You Want to Do

	Week 1	Week 2	Week 3	Week 4	Week 5
January					
February					
March					
April					
May					
June					
July					
August					
September					
October					
November					
December					

From *5K and 10K Training* by Brian Clarke, 2006, Champaign, IL: Human Kinetics.

racing too much and training too little. Constant racing is not a valid substitute for constant and progressive training.

Of course, you could rationalize frequent racing by "training through" your races. Training through a race is another way of saying you aren't tapering or recovering adequately. You should taper enough before your races to feel eager to race, and you should recover enough afterwards to be ready the next time you do a hard workout. That much resting can take a big hunk out of your training, especially when you race frequently. Thus, unless you are into a peaking period, you should curtail your urge to race.

During a sharpening period, however, you should race enough to know how your training is progressing. As you have seen, pace-specific training is tied to your current race pace. As long as you feel eager to race and you do a very hard racing effort, you can accept your race results as a valid indication of your current ability. Racing once every four to six weeks during a sharpening period should be enough for this purpose.

Develop a Training Program

At this juncture, I recommend drawing up a blank weekly calendar containing enough weeks to take you through your goal-race. Table 8.5 is an example of such a form, with enough space for planning a 15-week program. (You can download a longer form for free from my Web site at www.bcendurancetrainings.com.)

Table 8.5   Training and Racing Program

Week	Mon	Tues	Wed	Thu	Fri	Sat	Sun
1							
2							
3							
4							
5							
6							
7							
8							
9							
10							
11							
12							
13							
14							
15							

From *5K and 10K Training* by Brian Clarke, 2006, Champaign, IL: Human Kinetics.

Please begin the planning process by filling in table 8.5 with all the races you plan to run during the program, including your goal-race at the end of the program. This is your racing schedule, with the goal-race being the focal point of a training program you will soon develop.

Next, pencil in your weekly training schedule by indicating when and how hard you will train each week leading up to your goal-race. You'll recall from chapter 4 that a training schedule tells you when and how hard you will train during a training week. Indicate on table 8.5 whether a race or workout will be run in the a.m. or p.m., as well as its overall difficulty, whether easy (E), moderate (M), or hard (H).

You should have already drawn up a schedule in table 4.2. You could maintain that schedule or create a new schedule that provides you with options for running a new set of ability-building workouts. You'll plan those workouts a little later in this chapter. Now you should think in terms of how your schedule will change during the program. How many major and minor workouts will you do each week? How will the schedule change from period to period? How will it change as you taper for and recover from your races?

Notice whether your time off for tapering and recovering gives you adequate time to train. Count all your normal training weeks and compare that number with your weeks off for tapering and recovering. Unless you are planning a peaking/racing period, you should have at least a 3:1 ratio of training weeks to off-weeks. This is an opportunity to think critically about the number of practice races you are planning, and how they might complement or disrupt your training.

All you have at this point is a schedule of when you will race and when you will do your major and minor workouts. This is the framework within which your workouts will occur during the training program. You still haven't considered the ability-building purpose of those workouts.

Before you set up your workouts you should assess your racing ability. The goal is to build a full complement of abilities for your next goal-race. Because training time could be short, you should take advantage of abilities you already have by considering your current ability profile.

Assess Your Ability Profile

Your ability profile is based on the abilities you may have developed recently, including stamina, power, tempo, speed and endurance. The material in chapters 3 and 7 should have clarified the meaning of these words. So, given the training you have done in the past six months, what racing abilities do you possess?

Table 8.6 will answer this question by helping you to rate the racing abilities you've built with your three hardest weekly workouts and your recovery runs.

Table 8.6 Rating Racing Abilities from Hardest Recent Workouts

	No workout	Workout #1	Workout #2	Workout #3	Recovery runs
Stamina: The ability to run long and slow.					
Power: The ability to run uphill at a relaxed pace.					
Tempo: The ability to run comfortably at race pace.					
Speed: The ability to sprint or surge faster than race pace.					
Endurance: The ability to sustain uncomfortable race exertion.					

From *5K and 10K Training* by Brian Clarke, 2006, Champaign, IL: Human Kinetics.

Remember, all workouts build some ability, whether stamina, power, tempo, speed, or endurance. If you think about the meaning of each ability, you'll see which ones you may have built with your recent training. Notice that table 8.6 includes brief definitions of the five abilities.

Fill out table 8.6 by entering a number between 1 and 5 in the appropriate space. If, for example, your workout #1 is a fully developed, long and slow stamina run, put a "5" in the space on the stamina level in the workout #1 column. The number you'll enter for each workout represents the extent to which you have developed an ability, as indicated by the following scale. Note: If you haven't trained for an ability recently, put an appropriate number in the "No workout" column.

Nonexistent (1): You haven't trained for this ability at all. Nor does your natural ability lend itself to having this ability.

Rudimentary (2): You have this ability in small measure either because of some natural talent or because of some training in the past.

Partially Developed (3): You have trained for this ability in recent months, though inconsistently. Your ability is *passable*, but not effective.

Effectively Developed (4): You have trained consistently for this ability in recent months. You can use the ability *effectively* in your training and racing.

Fully Developed (5): You have trained consistently for this ability in recent months and you are *fully able* to use it in your training and racing.

You should end up with a rating for each ability listed in table 8.6. You should also see that your training is either stacked in favor of one or two abilities, or distributed evenly among most or all of them. On this basis you should have an idea of your ability profile and a sense of the abilities you may want to build for a coming goal-race.

Outline Your Training Program

Having rated your racing abilities, the main questions are, What abilities do you lack? Which ones should you continue building? And which ones can you overlook during this program because you have already built them?

It's difficult in a short-term program to build a full complement of racing abilities from scratch. So, take another look at your training and racing calendar. Try to envision the abilities you can build with the major workouts you have scheduled. Your major weekly workouts can each represent a separate ability-building progression. Given the number of weeks in your program and the number of workouts you will run each week, how many abilities can you reasonably expect to build?

Depending on the number of major workouts you will do each week, you may have several workout progressions to play with. These progressions will build the abilities you'll need for effective racing, including abilities that fill out your current repertoire. With each workout you propose to run, you should begin

INJURY AND PROGRAMMATIC RECOVERY

Recently, while sprinting away from some people at the finish of a race, I injured myself severely. I won the race with these competitors by limping the last 50 meters, but I paid the price of being in excruciating pain whenever I took a normal step for the next two weeks. Once I started walking "normally," I still had a minor limp. It took another week before I could resume training with very slow jogging. That's an extreme example, but it's also a case of how a severe injury can force a complete layoff.

Most minor injuries will go away with a few days of easy training, but chronic injuries are another problem. It's common to be chronically injured at the end of a training program. Chronic injuries are generally at the deep, dull ache level; they can cause minor limping during a run or at least some adjustments in stride or footfall. Chronic injuries are serious problems because they prevent proper running function and, thereby, often cause related injury problems. If you are chroni-

cally injured at the end of a program year, you should make your recovery period long enough and inactive enough to get over the injury completely. I've taken as many as three years off to get rid of serious chronic injuries. They were so intractable that I had begun to think I would never be injury-free again.

You'll probably want to do *something* while you are recovering from an injury, so what's appropriate? My rule is to do nothing that continues or renews the pain of chronic injury. If a very slow, 30-minute jog renews the pain, that's too much. Some injuries are so serious that a cure is only possible with easy walking. That's why I extend an offer to any injured athlete: As long as they are injured, they can train with my fitness walkers at no cost.

I've taken advantage of the walker group myself. Their workouts are too easy to count as "training" for me, but that's the point. The difficulty of the workout doesn't matter as long as I'm injured and need to walk *under* whatever pain I'm experiencing. I simply relax my competitive attitude and enjoy the walkers' company.

with a clear idea of its ability-building purpose. Will you build stamina, power, tempo, speed or endurance? Or will you build a combination of these abilities within a single workout?

Take some time to map out the purpose of each major workout progression, using table 8.5 to abbreviate the purpose of your workouts. You don't have to think about specific workout structures yet. Try instead to see how the progressions might develop chronologically. Keep in mind you'll need time to introduce and establish a workout without hurting yourself. The amount of time you'll need will depend in part on the similarity of recent workouts compared with the new workouts you aim to establish. If they are similar in structure, you can establish a new workout in relatively little time, say, a couple of weeks. Otherwise, it could take a month or more to introduce and establish the workout step-by-step.

You should also consider the approximate number of weeks you'll need to adapt to a workout. You may see some progress within several weeks, but the real issue is the amount of time it will take to become *fully able* to do the workout. Six weeks is not a long time to adapt completely to a new workout once you've established it.

So, given the amount of time you have between the start of the program and your goal-race, how many workouts can you reasonably expect to introduce sequentially? The answer to this question will tell you how many training periods you can fit into your program.

Plan Training Periods

Once you've adapted as much as possible to a workout, another workout could take its place. This new workout should be a continuation of an ongoing ability-building progression, but it will be situated within a new training period.

How many training periods can you reasonably fit within the program you are planning? In this book, I have presented a rationale for five periods: base building, sharpening, peaking, racing, and recovering. But you may not have time to develop different workout regimens for each of these periods. In that case, you'll have to streamline your program to meet your time frame.

It's okay to have only one training period within a program. And it's equally okay to begin with pace-specific workouts without a significant prior base of longer, slower training. You can always develop a traditional high-mileage base later when you have more time and your racing goals are not as urgent. Meanwhile, you should think in terms of making the best of an abbreviated program.

If time is short, you may have to run dual-purpose workouts within a single training period leading up to the goal-race. Given two or three parallel progressions within the same program, the various major workouts of each progression should complement one another in terms of purpose and structure. One workout could be a long run to provide the aerobic base for other shorter, faster workouts. Those other workouts could include pace-specific tempo, speed, and endurance intervals that build abilities you'll need for the goal-race.

If your program contains a single training period, you should think in terms of separate training phases within the period. First, you should allow yourself time to gradually phase in new workouts. Once a workout is established, you can think in terms of adapting to it during a second phase in which you repeat the workout, looking for improved performance. And as you approach your goal-race, you should think in terms of a tapering phase in which you decrease the frequency and overall effort of your workouts.

The goal of the taper phase is to be totally fresh and eager on race day. I generally work on the premise that nothing I do within the last two weeks will have a positive adaptive effect. Moreover, given the depth of fatigue associated with a weekly regimen of three hard workouts, two weeks is cutting it close for tapering. Thus, I recommend scheduling your last hard workout not later than three weeks before a goal-race and tapering your training from there.

At this point, you should have a good idea of the sort of progressions and the length of the training periods comprising your program. Next, you should think in terms of the particular workouts you will do, including their workout structures.

Set Up Your Workouts

Before you actually run a workout, you should set it up mentally. With each major workout you propose to run, you should begin with a clear idea of its ability-building purpose. Are you building stamina, power, tempo, speed, or endurance? Or are you building a combination of these abilities within a single workout? The purpose of the workout should give you an idea of its exertion structure, and how that heart rate structure builds a certain ability. If you need to review the basics, please refer to chapters 3 and 7.

Approximately what heart rate will you target to achieve your ability-building purpose? And how long should the workout be to keep your overall effort within your scheduled level (easy, moderate, or hard)? These are the two questions you should answer for yourself before you take your first running step. It might be a good idea to graph a workout before you run it. And while you are at it, you should also graph your hardest recent workout, comparing that workout with the one you are about to introduce.

One of the most important aspects of the setup process is deciding whether your new workout is within your current capacity for exertion. Earlier, you estimated the duration and the average level of exertion of your hardest current workout using figure 4.3. On the same form, please note the duration and average level of exertion of your proposed new workouts. If you aren't sure how to structure a new workout, feel free to use an appropriate workout from chapter 7. How do the old and new workouts compare?

Beware of jumping more than 15 or 20 heartbeats per minute without intermediate steps, or without a concurrent shortening of workout duration. Similarly, beware of adding a significant amount of time to a new workout without lowering your average level of exertion. In other words, based on what you are used to doing, is the new workout reasonably within your capacity? If the answer to this question is no, then you should moderate its exertion level and/or duration.

Taking the Next Step

The purpose of this chapter was to get you thinking about your personal running profile. Are you a recreational, competitive, or elite runner? When you get in shape, how fast are you? Are your racing goals currently more or less competitive or noncompetitive? Your profile determines the sort of training you will do within a program, whether basic or advanced.

A profile also includes the time you have to train before your goal-race. Most training programs are short enough to accommodate races coming up in six weeks to several months. I've made a case for thinking in terms of yearly programs that give you enough time to really develop a full complement of racing abilities. Yearly programs don't necessarily preclude racing effectively when you are in the middle of a training year. But you should give some thought to racing when you are at least fully adapted to the various workout regimens you schedule for yourself.

Remember, you must establish a regimen before you can gain adaptive value from it. Adaptation occurs when you repeat an established training stimulus at an optimal level. The next chapter will develop this idea by giving you ways to track your progress during a training program. More than a way of counting miles, an effective training log should give you a way of tracking your proficiency within the context of effort and energy.

CHAPTER 9

Tracking Your Progress

At this point, I have assembled the major concepts in this book of ideas. Virtually all of my ideas relate to the prime constructs of effort and energy. Given these ideas, I've suggested that you can use a variety of descriptive scales to measure changes in your capacity for exertion.

In an ideal world we would establish a regimen of workouts and train from week to week, building our ability until it reaches a peak on race day. Unfortunately, the real world is more complex than ideal. It's not always possible to detect a negative shift in ability until a significant trend has developed. Meanwhile, we spin our wheels doing workouts that could be maintaining our effectiveness at best, or leading us into significant inability at worst.

Thus, we have to pay close attention to measurable indications of effort, capacity, and performance. Since it isn't difficult to measure effort and performance, we can infer changes in capacity as long as we have a way of recording meaningful data. This chapter will describe an effort–energy training log and show you how to use it to measure changes in your proficiency.

Tracking Changes in Proficiency

Every workout affects your performance capacity in some way, whether positive, negative, or neutral. If minor changes occur from day to day, the cumulative effect on your capacity may take several weeks or more to become apparent. One reason to keep an effort–energy log is to discern these trends as soon as possible.

The main trends you are looking for relate to changes in your capacity for exertion. I've defined capacity in terms of energy, noting how it changes within a workout: *none, little, some, ample, abundant.* Or how it changes from day to day: *sluggish, tired, lazy, ready, eager.* Proficiency has to do with changes in your energy, too. But it is more precisely understood in terms of long-term changes in your ability to perform a race or workout.

For many years, the only way I could tell I was improving was by paying attention to my feelings of energy, strength, and confidence about the workouts I was running. I noticed that those feelings changed on the following scale: *unable, ineffective, passably able, effective,* and *fully able.* Even when improved performance was partly due to increased effort, I could tell I was getting stronger by noticing how much more effectively I could do a workout through a training period.

Eventually, however, I wanted to measure my proficiency more objectively. A few years ago, one of my athletes, Bjorn Marsen, a postdoctoral researcher in physics at the University of Hawaii, gave me a simple method. He defined proficiency as the measure of our ability to cover distance using yards per heartbeat as an objective standard. I'll describe how to calculate proficiency later in this chapter. Here you should know that it involves several simple spreadsheet calculations. All you supply is an average heart rate and your time for a known distance. The result is the average distance in yards (or meters) that you cover every time your heart beats.

A typical proficiency value is 1.123 yards per heartbeat (yds/hb). Since heart rates differ from person to person, proficiency values are not directly comparable among different athletes. In general, though, the fastest and most talented athletes cover more ground per heartbeat than slower, less talented athletes. Five- to six-hour marathoners, for instance, usually have proficiency ratings in the 0.850 to 0.950 range, while four-hour marathoners have readings in the 1.350 to 1.550 range. The fastest Hawaii athletes I've assessed are above 2.150 yds/hb.

Yet, knowing one's proficiency in relation to other runners is immaterial. One reason for calculating proficiency is to track the way your performance capacity changes within and between training programs. For instance, proficiency ratings for a recurring race event can show you how your year-round training has affected your ability in that particular race (see figure 9.1).

Measuring and Calculating Proficiency

You wouldn't be able to measure your proficiency without a heart rate monitor that has an average heart rate feature. The simplest POLAR heart rate monitor captures an average heart rate reading from the time you start the monitor to the time you stop it. The more complex monitors add the capability of averaging your heart rate for intervals within a workout.

Measuring proficiency also requires that you know your time and distance so you can calculate your pace in minutes per mile. The distance calculation doesn't

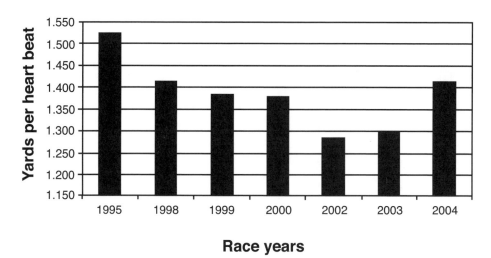

Figure 9.1 My proficiency decreased markedly after 1995, as indicated by my results for the Norman Tamanaha 15K. A chronic case of bursitis between 1996 and 2000 kept me from training effectively. After two years off, I finally began to train consistently again in 2003 with a slight upturn in my condition, which continued more dramatically with the 2004 race.

have to be exact. You could measure a course with an automobile odometer to get an approximation of the distance you have covered. Or you could make an educated guess at the distance. As long as you repeat the same course from workout to workout, it doesn't matter exactly how far you say it is. All that matters is the consistency of using the same distance for the same course every time you calculate your proficiency.

Some recovery runs might be a staple part of a training regimen, regardless of the training period. By measuring proficiency for those workouts, you can track your capacity through the various phases of a training cycle to see how it changes from training period to training period (see figure 9.2).

This tracking process enables you to measure changes in your performance capacity. Given such accurate and objective benchmarks of your ability to perform, you can decide how to adjust your training to accommodate your body's adaptive cycles.

There are several steps to calculating proficiency. It helps to do these calculations on a computer with a spreadsheet program such as Microsoft Excel. Table 9.1 is a replica of a spreadsheet I use to calculate proficiency for a 3.74-mile recovery run. As I enter the number of minutes and seconds it took to run the workout in the "Min" and "Sec" columns, a hidden formula in the "Time" column computes my time in minutes. Using my time and the known distance of the workout, the hidden formula in the "Pace" column calculates my pace automatically. Then, once I add my average heart rate in the "HR" column, hidden formulas in the last two columns calculate my proficiency (as yards per heart beat) for the workout.

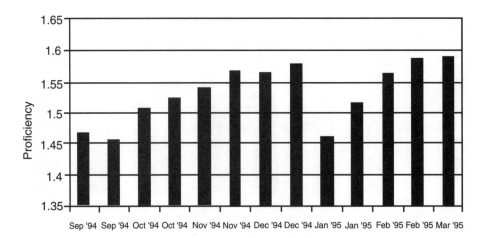

(Each bar represents the two-week average for 3.75-mile recovery run)

Figure 9.2   This bar graph shows my proficiency during two training periods: a 16-week base-building period and a subsequent 10-week peaking period. Each bar represents my proficiency, averaged during two-week miniperiods for the same easy run. The graph shows that my ability went through successive phases of shock, adaptation, and exhaustion.

Table 9.1   Calculating Proficiency With a Spreadsheet Program

Min	Sec	HR	Time	Pace	Beats/mile	Yds/beat
40	18	109	40.30	10.8	1,175	1.498
41	00	108	41.00	11.0	1,184	1.487
41	00	113	41.00	11.0	1,239	1.421
38	14	110	38.23	10.2	1,125	1.565
38	34	109	38.57	10.3	1,124	1.566
38	31	110	38.52	10.3	1,133	1.554
38	00	106	38.00	10.2	1,077	1.634

Using a spreadsheet program, all you need to do is enter your time (in minutes and seconds) for a workout, as well as your average heart rate. The computer does everything else automatically so you can immediately see your proficiency reading. Otherwise, you'll have to make your calculations laboriously with a calculator according to the following procedure:

> **Calculate your total time in seconds.** You should have a total time for a race, workout, or interval recorded in your training log. It will look something like

TRACKING PROFICIENCY

I have used the proficiency calculation to track my ability in the annual Norman Tamanaha Memorial 15K. I ran 61:30 for the race as a 51-year-old in April, 1995. While that time was more than nine minutes slower than I had run in 1979, I was happy with my 1995 performance because I was well-prepared. I had run 70-mile training weeks through the previous fall. As a result, my proficiency reading for the 1995 race was 1.521 yds/hb (see figure 9.1 on page 149).

In the months before the 1999 Tamanaha 15K, by contrast, my average weekly mileage was less than 40. I was suffering from a serious case of bursitis—the same condition I'd had off and on since rupturing my Achilles bursa in the mid-80s. The pain had kept me from building a solid base of stamina. Although I ran the 1999 Tamanaha 15K more than a minute faster than I had in 1998, my average heart rate increased from 176 to 183 BPM. That increase in heart rate lowered my proficiency to 1.382 yds/hb, the equivalent of 25 yards per minute slower than I had run the 1995 race.

It had taken an all-out effort on my part to be competitive in the 1999 15K, but I was faking my ability because I hadn't trained well the previous year; in fact, I wasn't in good condition. In 2000, I ran the Tamanaha 15K again in the same time I'd achieved in 1999, but my average heart rate rose one beat per minute and my proficiency dropped accordingly. With that all-out performance, I had tapped out my ability to muscle the race with effort. My proficiency was down to 1.375 yds/hb, and I was too injured to train effectively. Knowing this, I shut my training down completely

for the first time in five years to focus on healing the bursitis.

During the next two years, I did no hard training, maintaining minimal fitness by jogging and walking with the slower athletes in my training programs. On the basis of that regimen, I ran the Tamanaha 15K again in 2002, with a time of 70:33 and an average heart rate of 181 BPM, which gave me a proficiency of 1.282—a personal nadir for the race. In 2003, I ran the Tamanaha 15K as a hard workout rather than a race because I didn't want to risk reinjury. I had spent most of the previous year recovering from injuries related to the weakened condition of my feet and an overly ambitious comeback schedule. I ran 81 minutes for the race and my heart rate averaged 155 BPM, which gave me a proficiency of 1.296—slightly improved from the 1.282 of the previous year. I was injury-free and determined not to reinjure myself, but I was extremely fragile.

During 2003, I noticed that any running in the 140 to 150 BPM range (low to mid-steady state) was either risky or downright injurious. On that basis I decided to set a heart rate limit of 130 BPM on all of my workouts. I also decided to avoid steep hills, intervals, and long runs. My staple workout was a moderate six-mile run from my home on most mornings. I enjoyed the run through a moderately hilly valley in the early morning shade of a steep adjoining ridge.

Though I was tempted to slip into longer runs, I discovered that the shorter runs were working. I was staying injury-free and I was getting stronger, a feeling that was confirmed during the 2004 Tamanaha 15K when my proficiency rose to 1.412 yds/hb. I was on the way back and having fun with my training.

4:18, 68:12 or 2:05:48. The basic formula for converting these times to seconds is (hours × 60 × 60) + (minutes × 60) + (seconds) equals your total time in seconds. Two hours, five minutes, and 48 seconds is computed as

$$(2 \times 60 \times 60 = 7{,}200) + (5 \times 60 = 300) + 48 = 7{,}548 \text{ seconds}$$

> **Calculate your pace in minutes per mile.** Once you have your total time in seconds, you can calculate your pace in minutes per mile. Divide your time in seconds by the number of miles in the workout. If you ran an 11.5 mile workout in 7,548 seconds, for instance, the calculation would be

$$7{,}548/11.5 = 656 \text{ seconds per mile}$$

$$656/60 = 10.9 \text{ minutes per mile}$$

> **Calculate your average heartbeats per mile.** Take your pace in minutes per mile and multiply it by your average heart rate. For example, if your pace is 10.9 minutes per mile and your average heart rate is 130 BPM,

$$10.9 \times 130 = 1{,}417, \text{ which is the average number of heartbeats per mile during the workout}$$

> **Calculate your proficiency.** Divide 1,760 (the number of yards in a mile) by the number of beats per mile to get the number of yards you ran per heartbeat.

$$1{,}760/1{,}417 = 1.242 \text{ yards per heartbeat}$$

In this example, the figure 1.242 could be your base level of proficiency for a workout. If you were to improve your proficiency by 0.25 yards per heartbeat, you would be running nine inches farther every time your heart beat. If your average heart rate for the workout is 130 beats per minute, then

$$9 \times 130 = 1{,}170 \text{ inches, or } 97.5 \text{ feet, per minute that you are running farther than you were at your base level.}$$

Sighting Signs of Adaptation

I often do my intervals, looking for signs of adaptation. Typically, my heart rate readings level out about two-thirds of the way through an interval workout. Sometimes at that point my times continue to drop slightly at the same heart rate, and I wonder whether I'm seeing an adaptive shift in my ability. It's difficult to tell what's going on in the moment, though, because heart rate readings are constantly shifting on the face of the monitor.

Nonetheless, I've learned to feel small increases in proficiency: a slight relaxing of my body despite the onset of fatigue and an increased flow of energy that's reminiscent of a second wind. These feelings of sustained ability never last longer than a few intervals, but I can usually confirm them later once I've put my pace and heart rate data into the computer (see table 9.2). This table shows that proficiency drops until the fifth interval. Then, with average heart rate holding at the 150 bpm level, proficiency rises slightly during the sixth and seventh intervals. This slight rise in proficiency is difficult to detect from looking at a

Table 9.2   Signs of Adaptation Within an Interval Workout

	Average HR	Interval time	Proficiency
1	130	7:35	1.785
2	139	7:30	1.688
3	143	7:21	1.675
4	147	7:18	1.640
5	150	7:19	1.604
6	150	7:18	**1.607**
7	150	7:15	**1.618**
8	153	7:21	1.565

monitor during a workout, but it becomes apparent when pace and heart rate data are subsequently computed.

I know I should end the workout when I notice that my pace has slowed at the same easy, flowing effort. I may be able to continue running, but any further increment of adaptive value will be more than offset by a debilitating increase in fatigue.

Sometimes, I speed up during a workout looking for signs of adaptation. This speed-up tendency is a completely irrational habit held over from the days when the only way I could prove I was getting stronger was to run faster. Calculating proficiency using pace and heart rate data sidestepped this inanity, because forcing my times down no longer worked. In fact, the proficiency calculation guarantees that a faster time will be offset by a corresponding increase in exertion, leaving proficiency unaffected.

Nonetheless, it is possible to be deceived by one's proficiency readings. Ordinarily, heart rate increases in direct proportion to increases in pace. Above a certain level of exertion, however, increases in pace will result in proportionally smaller increases in heart rate. Under these circumstances, your proficiency would appear to increase, say, at the end of a steady-state interval workout when, for the fun of it, you've taken your exertion up to ragged edge. This is a false increase because, in fact, proficiency decreases as fatigue sets in.

This principle is something for you keep in mind when you are comparing intervals, races, or workouts at drastically different levels of exertion. It's like comparing apples to oranges. Thus, it's okay to compare performances at comparable levels of exertion, either high or low, but comparing drastically different levels will give you a false impression of your proficiency.

Another way you can be deceived by a proficiency reading is when you are comparing workouts with different levels of energy. If you are tracking your proficiency for an easy recovery run, for instance, you should only compare times and heart rate readings where your workout energy was the same. In other words, an easy/tired workout is not the same as an easy/lazy workout because your capacity for exertion is not the same in both cases.

Remember, your capacity is your metabolic engine. The more energy you have the greater your engine, and the faster you can run with less effort. Keep this principle in mind when you are sorting and grouping workouts and races for comparison using the proficiency calculation.

MEASURING ADAPTATION

During the fall of 1994, I managed to build my weekly mileage from 50 to 70 by adding double workouts to my regimen and by slowing down dramatically on all of my runs. (I wrote about this training regimen in *Running by Feeling*, published by *Competitive Running Press* in 1999.)

One of my goals was to measure adaptive changes garnered with my high-mileage training regimen. During the first six weeks of the training period, my times for my easy 3.74-mile recovery run were an average of 43 minutes—considerably slower than a previous, low-mileage average of 36 minutes. Generally, my energy for these runs was terrible. I was usually tired, and only after six weeks did I begin to feel lazy for most of the recovery runs.

I hung in at 70 miles a week for 16 weeks, keeping careful heart rate records of all my recovery runs. Since I averaged 10 recovery runs a week, I reasoned that my performances on those runs would serve as statistically significant benchmarks for changes in my ability. In addition to my

easy recovery runs, I was doing a long run, an interval workout, and a hill run. Those workouts would contribute to my overall condition, which in turn would manifest itself in my ability to do the recovery runs. I kept track of my average heart rate and ran the workouts on the same 3.74-mile course.

When my times varied for the easy run, they did so according to how much energy I had. The better I felt, the faster I ran. I averaged 36 minutes on the two occasions when I felt ready; and I averaged 43 minutes when I was sluggish. Most of the time I was lazy for the easy runs, and my average time for those workouts was 39 minutes. For purposes of measuring adaptation, I decided that I should only compare apples with apples, so I looked at easy/lazy workouts where I averaged 109 beats per minute.

I had run eight of those workouts during the 16-week training period, and my times had dropped steadily from 44 minutes in early September to 38 minutes in early December. I decided this performance progression was a manifestation of adaptation.

Maintaining an Effort–Energy Log

I developed a training log years ago as a way to keep track of my personal training. I soon realized that the log would also serve as a way for the runners in my marathon training programs to communicate with me about their training.

I had 60 athletes training under my direction for the 2004 Honolulu Marathon. They ranged in ability from seven-hour walkers to four-hour runners. These athletes were divided into six distinct groups of runners, joggers, and walkers, each of whom had a separate group leader and different courses to do whenever we met to train. Obviously, I couldn't be with each group during every workout, so the training logs were useful to me for handling training problems before they could become acute. I read the logs between workouts and followed up with certain athletes, often to learn more about an injury and to come to an agreement about how to deal with it.

My Personal Training Diary

As for my own running, I keep the log on my dresser at home where I can see it immediately after every workout. The idea is to record the basic data for a workout as soon as possible after running it. If I let a day or two slip before recording a workout, I'll forget my experience of effort and energy. All those easy morning and evening workouts seem to blend together after a while. Yet, in the moment, they are unique activities with distinct effort and energy patterns.

The only time I don't keep the log is when I'm sick or injured and not training. In my frustration with a cold or injury I feel as though there is nothing of substance to record. Once I've decided to resume training, however, and once I've recorded several workouts, keeping the log quickly becomes a habit and a part of my training discipline. It's also a momentum builder. I like to see my mileage accumulate during

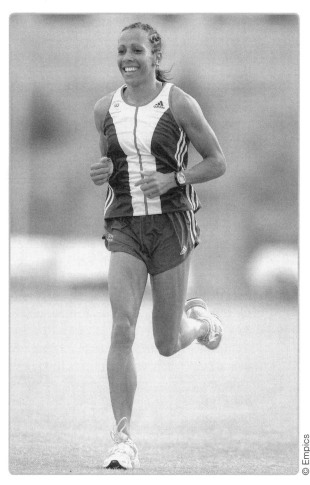

© Empics

There are no hard, fast rules when it comes to running workouts. But generally it's better to enjoy a workout than to abhor its difficulty.

the week, and I like having the awareness that filling out the effort and energy scales gives me.

I believe that having my athletes fill out the log helps them with their awareness, too. They come into training thinking in terms of pace and mileage, but they soon learn to think in terms of effort and energy. For example, the joggers begin to see that their slow pace is the same as the runners' slow pace, even though the runners are running faster. After all, both groups are breathing conversationally. Similarly, both groups run for two hours, but the runner group goes several miles farther. That doesn't mean the joggers should run longer to make up the mileage shortfall. After all, both groups ran hard workouts.

I used to have the joggers in my marathon programs run as far as the runners. But the joggers ended up on the road a lot longer than the runners, which was discouraging for them. Worse, the joggers ended up getting injured and exhausted, and many of them did poorly in the marathon, if they even made it to the starting line. Now, I have the joggers do a long run of about 14 miles in three hours, which is the same time as the better runners take to do 20 miles. The joggers do a five- or six-hour marathon and enjoy the event, which is what they wanted in the first place.

Despite the folklore about needing to do a certain number of miles in training, there are no hard and fast rules or formulas for distance running. Much of what we learn happens from our experience. What you should be looking for are training patterns that lead to successful races. If you discover, for example, that you race well when you taper down to 25 miles the week before a race, then that's good information. For others, however, 25 miles may represent their top weekly mileage so tapering to 12 miles might be better for them.

We have to consider individual circumstances, even when generalizing about joggers or runners. Some people prefer to leave these issues to a coach or trainer; others like to figure out their own patterns. The best way to see those patterns is to keep a training and racing log, and by reading that record from time to time with pertinent questions in mind. In this regard, a log serves much more effectively than memory. Memory is selective and deteriorates with time; the log tells you closely and accurately what you were experiencing on a particular date.

In order to obtain accurate information, you must be honest with yourself. It won't help when you can't recall whether your mileage total for a week was a gross exaggeration because you were trying to impress yourself at the time. Similarly, it's easy to delude yourself about being injured for a workout. Sometimes, I fudge my mileage or overlook a persistent pain to make myself feel better in the moment. But this is a form of lying or cheating, which ultimately detracts from my self-esteem. Thus, I generally assume a resolutely honest attitude in filling out the log so I can accurately reflect my training experience.

Ultimately, the log is the barebones story of your training and racing. Naturally, you'll embellish the story in the telling, but you've got to have the basic facts in hand if you want to analyze your training for the purpose of making it better.

Filling Out the Log

The effort–energy training log shown in figure 9.3 enables you to record the fundamental experiential data of a workout. You can also access a free version from my Web site at www.bcendurancetrainings.com.

  The following instructions for filling out the log and the accompanying definitions of the terms will come in handy for understanding how to complete it. In order to make effective use of the log, you have to understand the meaning of the words, especially the distinctions between levels of the scales. Until you familiarize yourself with the language of adaptive training, you'll continue having difficulty filling out the diary. You should be conversant in each term and each level so eventually you will know how to fill out the log to describe your running accurately.

  The following questions and definitions will help you to understand the log, as well as focus on important aspects of your training.

1. Workout effort: How hard was the workout *as a whole?*

   > Very Easy: Very short and very slow; you recover in less than 12 hours.

   > Easy: Short and slow; 12-hour recovery needed.

   > Moderate: Intermediate tempo and duration; 24- to 30-hour recovery; some fatigue, but hardly noticeable.

   > Hard: Noticeably fatiguing workout; 48 to 60 hours for recovery.

   > Very Hard: Very fatiguing; more than 60 hours for recovery.

   > All-Out: Couldn't have run faster for the distance or farther without slowing down. You need one day of recovery for every all-out/eager racing mile.

2. Workout energy: What pattern of energy developed during the workout?

   > Sluggish: No energy developed during the workout.

   > Tired: Little energy developed, and it ran out early.

   > Lazy: Some energy developed after a long warm-up, but it was insufficient for a hard workout.

   > Ready: Ample energy developed after a short warm-up, and it was sufficient for a hard workout.

   > Eager: Abundant energy developed quickly, and it was sufficient for a racing effort. You have an aggressive attitude.

3. Attitude regarding effort: What was your attitude about the effort of the workout?

   > Oppressed: Unpleasant, detestable drudgery.

   > Burdened: Duty bound to perform, no pleasure, wearisome.

   > Satisfied: Pleasant, okay; neither positive nor negative.

   > Enjoyed: Pleasurable, delightful, or fun.

   > Exhilarated: Feeling of supreme well-being, including mild euphoria.

Figure 9.3

Effort–Energy Training Log

Date: am pm	Workout:		Duration:	Mileage workout/cum:	
Workout effort:	Very easy	Easy	Moderate	Hard	Very hard
Workout energy:	Sluggish - 0 +	Tired - 0 +	Lazy - 0 +	Ready - 0 +	Eager - 0 +
Attitude re effort:	Oppressed	Burdened	Satisfied	Enjoyed	Exhilarated
Workout pain:	Tender	Twinge	Ache	Sore	Severe
Life energy:	Exhausted	Weary	Able to work	Rested	Energetic
Comments:					
Heart rate data:					

Date: am pm	Workout:		Duration:	Mileage workout/cum:	
Workout effort:	Very easy	Easy	Moderate	Hard	Very hard
Workout energy:	Sluggish - 0 +	Tired - 0 +	Lazy - 0 +	Ready - 0 +	Eager - 0 +
Attitude re effort:	Oppressed	Burdened	Satisfied	Enjoyed	Exhilarated
Workout pain:	Tender	Twinge	Ache	Sore	Severe
Life energy:	Exhausted	Weary	Able to work	Rested	Energetic
Comments:					
Heart rate data:					

Date: am pm	Workout:		Duration:	Mileage workout/cum:	
Workout effort:	Very easy	Easy	Moderate	Hard	Very hard
Workout energy:	Sluggish - 0 +	Tired - 0 +	Lazy - 0 +	Ready - 0 +	Eager - 0 +
Attitude re effort:	Oppressed	Burdened	Satisfied	Enjoyed	Exhilarated
Workout pain:	Tender	Twinge	Ache	Sore	Severe
Life energy:	Exhausted	Weary	Able to work	Rested	Energetic
Comments:					
Heart rate data:					

Date: am pm	Workout:		Duration:	Mileage workout/cum:	
Workout effort:	Very easy	Easy	Moderate	Hard	Very hard
Workout energy:	Sluggish - 0 +	Tired - 0 +	Lazy - 0 +	Ready - 0 +	Eager - 0 +
Attitude re effort:	Oppressed	Burdened	Satisfied	Enjoyed	Exhilarated
Workout pain:	Tender	Twinge	Ache	Sore	Severe
Life energy:	Exhausted	Weary	Able to work	Rested	Energetic
Comments:					
Heart rate data:					

From *5K and 10K Training* by Brian Clarke, 2006, Champaign, IL: Human Kinetics.

Effort–Energy Training Log (*continued*)

Date: am pm	Workout:		Duration:	Mileage workout/cum:	
Workout effort:	Very easy	Easy	Moderate	Hard	Very hard
Workout energy:	Sluggish - 0 +	Tired - 0 +	Lazy - 0 +	Ready - 0 +	Eager - 0 +
Attitude re effort:	Oppressed	Burdened	Satisfied	Enjoyed	Exhilarated
Workout pain:	Tender	Twinge	Ache	Sore	Severe
Life energy:	Exhausted	Weary	Able to work	Rested	Energetic
Comments:					
Heart rate data:					

Date: am pm	Workout:		Duration:	Mileage workout/cum:	
Workout effort:	Very easy	Easy	Moderate	Hard	Very hard
Workout energy:	Sluggish - 0 +	Tired - 0 +	Lazy - 0 +	Ready - 0 +	Eager - 0 +
Attitude re effort:	Oppressed	Burdened	Satisfied	Enjoyed	Exhilarated
Workout pain:	Tender	Twinge	Ache	Sore	Severe
Life energy:	Exhausted	Weary	Able to work	Rested	Energetic
Comments:					
Heart rate data:					

Date: am pm	Workout:		Duration:	Mileage workout/cum:	
Workout effort:	Very easy	Easy	Moderate	Hard	Very hard
Workout energy:	Sluggish - 0 +	Tired - 0 +	Lazy - 0 +	Ready - 0 +	Eager - 0 +
Attitude re effort:	Oppressed	Burdened	Satisfied	Enjoyed	Exhilarated
Workout pain:	Tender	Twinge	Ache	Sore	Severe
Life energy:	Exhausted	Weary	Able to work	Rested	Energetic
Comments:					
Heart rate data:					

Date: am pm	Workout:		Duration:	Mileage workout/cum:	
Workout effort:	Very easy	Easy	Moderate	Hard	Very hard
Workout energy:	Sluggish - 0 +	Tired - 0 +	Lazy - 0 +	Ready - 0 +	Eager - 0 +
Attitude re effort:	Oppressed	Burdened	Satisfied	Enjoyed	Exhilarated
Workout pain:	Tender	Twinge	Ache	Sore	Severe
Life energy:	Exhausted	Weary	Able to work	Rested	Energetic
Comments:					
Heart rate data:					

From *5K and 10K Training* by Brian Clarke, 2006, Champaign, IL: Human Kinetics.

EFFORT–ENERGY LOG INSTRUCTIONS

Here's how to fill out the log:

> Date: Enter the number of the month and day (for example, August 26 is written as 8-26). Circle "a.m.," "noon" or "p.m." to indicate when you ran the workout.

> Workout: Enter a brief description of the workout—just enough to know what the workout was or what course you ran. Note: Further workout details go in the comments section of the form.

> Duration: Enter your time from the start to the finish of the workout in minutes (up to 120 minutes). If the workout was more than 120 minutes, enter hours and minutes (for example, 2:20 for two hours and 20 minutes).

> Mileage (workout/cum): Enter two numbers with a slash between them to indicate the number of miles in the workout and the cumulative number of miles for the week.

> Workout effort: Circle the appropriate option. You can fine-tune these entries by circling the plus, minus, or zero sign. For example, if a workout was more difficult than an easy workout but not quite moderate, check the easy box and circle the plus sign.

> Workout energy: First, check the pattern of energy that developed during the workout. Then determine whether that pattern was more or less than standard (the zero sign), circling the appropriate plus or minus sign.

> Attitude regarding effort: Check the lowest level that reflects your attitude about the effort of the workout as you were running it.

> Workout pain: Leave this scale blank if you were not injured. Otherwise, check the appropriate option. Enter the location of the injury in the comments section.

> Life energy: Check the lowest level that reflects your ability to function in life *between* this workout and the last workout.

> Comments: Enter any relevant details regarding the workout: routes, split or interval times, insights, concerns, and problems.

4. Workout pain: How badly were you injured? (Don't mark if not injured.)

   > Tender: Nonspecific discomfort.

   > Twinge: Darting pain with each step.

   > Ache: Chronic burning pain; deep and dull.

   > Sore: Major injury; causes limping.

   > Severe: Too painful to run on.

5. Life energy: How did you feel at work and at home since your last hard workout? (Record the *lowest* you felt.)

   > Exhausted: Nonfunctional; must go to sleep.

   > Weary: Stressed out; irritable and badly in need of a nap.

   > Able: Can function at work or play, but not cheerfully.

   > Rested: Good energy through the day, but you fall asleep early.

   > Energetic: Good energy through the day and evening.

I recommend copying the above definitions for easy reference and pasting them into the back cover of your log binder. Once you understand the concepts, you can use them effectively to measure your workout experience.

The notes you enter in your log are raw data. In order to convert that data into meaningful information, you've got to understand it in context with the training process. It's not enough, for instance, to know that you ran a hard/lazy workout or that you were burdened by the workout effort.

It should occur to you, for instance, that a hard/lazy workout is potentially exhaustive. You should also know how to weigh and evaluate the relative adaptive value of running hard/lazy versus moderate/lazy. Understanding how a hard/lazy workout could affect your performance capacity, you'll be able to make intelligent and necessary training decisions.

Whether a disharmonious effort is an indication of serious dysfunction depends on whether it's an anomaly or part of a recurring practice. Practices develop into metabolic trends because every workout affects your capacity in some way—whether positive, negative, or neutral. If minor changes occur from day to day, the cumulative effect on performance capacity may take several weeks or more to become apparent. One reason to keep an effort–energy log is to discern these trends with alacrity.

Tracking Training Patterns

Tracking mileage is one of the time-honored ways to determine how well you are running. The log has space for the mileage of each workout, in addition to a cumulative weekly total. I count my miles from Sunday morning to Saturday evening and circle the weekly total for easy reference. Then I graph my weekly mileage so I can see one week in relation to the others during a training period and within a program year.

You can download a mileage form for free from my Web site (www.bcendurance-trainings.com). If you keep the mileage form at the back of your training log, you can conveniently enter your mileage at the completion of a training week. It only takes a moment to update the form and, because it is a graphic representation of your mileage, you can see how one week relates to others during a training period.

The goal is to be as consistent as possible with regard to mileage. In the real world, however, work and family duties along with injuries and other stress symptoms can force us to adjust our mileage while preventing us from being as consistent as we would like. Moreover, the human mind tends to forget pertinent details, like the weeks when our mileage dropped because of injury. This mileage form will give you a visual way of measuring your weekly mileage so you can see at a glance how well you are following planned and gradual programmatic increases.

Seeing a pattern of gradually increasing mileage can be highly motivating. I find myself looking forward to making that weekly entry and figuratively patting myself on the back for another job well done. There is no question that race performance is ultimately related to weekly mileage, so there's nothing wrong with making mileage a strong motivating factor in our training. On the other hand, too much mileage can lead to injury, illness, and exhaustion. Thus, we also need a way to visualize our energy in relation to our mileage.

I've made the point that effort and energy are the building blocks of adaptation. In order to build ability, we have to coordinate our efforts with our energy as we train from day-to-day. I've already illustrated effort and energy in this book, using circles for effort and curves for energy (see figure 4.1). In my own training, I find it useful sometimes to track my effort and energy in a visual format, drawing circles and curves on a blank form. It would be nice to have a computer do the work of illustrating our effort and energy. Someday, no doubt, we will have a program for that purpose. Meanwhile, you will have to take the time to draw circles and curves on a blank form

You can download a version of this form from my Web site, www.bcendurance-trainings.com. I use a simple plastic ruler as a template for drawing circles on the form. I let the smallest circle represent very easy workouts, with increasingly larger circles representing the other workout effort levels. My training log tells me how hard each race or workout was, so I read the log and draw in the circles in the appropriate time slots on the form. Then I draw in the energy curves according to the level of workout energy I recorded in my log, using the workout energy scale on the form as a guide for the height of the curves.

With six weeks of training represented graphically on a single page, it's easy to see trends developing. Lots of large effort circles, for instance, lead to lower-level energy curves. In fact, lots of effort circles of any size can lead to lower-level energy curves. This isn't rocket science, especially in this visual medium. Overtraining leads to exhaustion; it's as simple as that. But seeing it in graphic form can have a powerful effect on one's way of thinking. We're apt to say, "Oh, too much effort *does* have a negative effect on my energy."

Once a month or so, I download the data from my heart rate monitor to my computer. At the same time, I enter data from my training log to a spreadsheet file. I already showed you part of this file in a previous section on proficiency. In addition to pace and heart rate data, I enter information about the effort and energy of the workout. That basic data leads to a summary sheet that tells a lot about my training for the month. I tally the following information:

> **Mileage.** This includes weekly mileage and average weekly mileage for the month. Mileage also includes average miles for hard, easy, and moderate workouts within an ability-building progression.

> **Workouts.** This includes the total number of workouts for the period, the average number of workouts per week, and the average number of hard, moderate, and easy workouts per week.

> **Effort.** Effort in this respect includes the average effort level per week (each workout effort has a number assigned to it according to its level: very easy = 1; easy = 2; moderate = 3; etc.). Add the effort level for all workouts in a week and divide by the number of workouts.

> **Energy.** Energy includes the average energy level per week (each energy level has a number assigned to it: sluggish = 1; tired = 2; lazy = 3; ready = 4; and eager = 5). Add the energy levels for all workouts in a week and divide by the number of workouts.

> **Effort/energy combinations.** There are thirty possible combinations, most of which are highly improbable. I keep track of the ones I actually run, tallying the number of optimal (harmonious) combinations and the number of nonoptimal (disharmonious) combinations.

> **Ability-building workout.** This includes the number of long runs per week, the number of tempo workouts per week, the number of hill runs per week, and the number of easy recovery runs per week.

It's interesting to see how this information changes from week to week and month to month. Again, I look for consistency in mileage, number of workouts, average effort and energy, and, of course, harmony between my effort and energy.

Taking the Next Step

This chapter described an effort–energy training log and showed you how to use it to measure changes in your proficiency. Proficiency is the measure of your ability to cover distance in yards per heart rate. This is one of the most important and useful ideas in this book. Used correctly, proficiency calculations can tell you when to continue a workout regimen or when to end it and begin another. It's easy to continue doing a set of workouts because you enjoy doing them, when from a competitive perspective you should quit doing that regimen because you are no longer gaining ability from it.

Remember, your training results are governed by shock, adaptation, and exhaustion. It's entirely possible that you could have ceased adapting to a training regimen, yet you don't show any of the classic signs of overtraining. You've simply reached an adaptive plateau and your times have stopped improving. Of course, it's okay to linger on an adaptive plateau, and to even race well at that level for some years. If you are frustrated with that scenario, however, there is hope. You can always train programmatically and progressively, and you can always gain more ability this year than last.

Epilogue

Throughout this book, I've spoken to you as an errant athlete needing wise counsel from an omnipotent expert. I realize, however, that no single reader could possibly warrant every admonition in this book. I also know that I'm hardly omnipotent when it comes to 5K and 10K training. In fact, I've made every mistake I write about in this book, which qualifies me as an errant athlete, too.

Competitive running is a difficult game to master. Yet, the difficulties of the sport only arise when winning and performance become important to us. At that point, our training becomes an issue and we have to think about the basic problems of the training process, among them building racing ability, scheduling workouts, and optimizing training effort. As complex as these problems are, the solutions are simple compared with subjects like nuclear physics.

The game of endurance athletics is mostly about patience and discipline. Athletes who do well in the sport are generally those who have outgrown their urge to race every workout. Though definitely a young person's game, the fastest runners are usually smart enough to have solved the recurrent problems or fortunate enough, as I was, to have had good coaches and teachers.

Ultimately, we are all coaching ourselves and learning from our particular experiences. In this sense, competitive running is a mental game as much as a physical one. In the final analysis, each of us has to think about our running in order to be successful at it. I hope this book has provided you with reasonable coaching and teaching alternatives.

Glossary

ability: Your capacity to perform in a race or workout.

adaptation: A long-term increase in your capacity for exertion. Greater capacity enables you to run faster and/or longer with the same effort.

adaptive plateau: A stabilizing of capacity to perform at a level that's usually somewhat lower than peak proficiency.

adaptive value: The potential of an effort/energy combination for increasing your capacity for exertion.

all-out effort: The point where fatigue forces you to run slower than your average pace for a given workout or racing distance.

anaerobic threshold: The point at which breathing becomes audible and heavy. During a hard/ready workout, threshold exertion is usually a range between 80 and 89 percent of maximum heart rate.

capacity for exertion: Capacity is the limit within which you can exert an effort, as well as the energy necessary to exert it.

consistency: The quality of different effort/energy combinations. As effort or energy changes so does consistency.

double workouts: Training twice a day.

effort: A generic term that encompasses two major constructs: pace exertion and workout effort.

effort/energy combination: One of 30 ways you can experience effort and energy during a race or workout.

endurance: The ability to endure uncomfortable race exertion.

energy: A generic term that refers to two major constructs: running energy and workout energy.

energy cycle: The ebb and flow of running energy as it changes from the start of one workout to the start of the next.

exertion: The effort necessary to generate a running pace, couched in terms of heart rate, breathing, power, tempo, and intensity.

exertion level: One of six distinctive ways of experiencing the exertion necessary to generate a progressively faster running pace.

exertion structure: The graphic configuration of your heart rate from start to finish of a race or workout.

exhaustion: A long-term decrease in capacity for exertion that reduces racing ability.

fatigue: A short-term decrease in capacity for exertion, generally associated with having some, little, or no running energy.

goal-race: The central, ability-building focus of a training program.

hard–easy system: The process of coordinating workout effort with different levels of workout energy to increase the likelihood of improved and satisfying race performance.

intensity: The degree of discomfort associated with the buildup of lactic acid and fatigue in the second half of a race or workout.

optimum effort: An effort exerted in harmony with the pattern of energy that develops during a race or workout.

overtraining: The activity of exerting too much effort during a workout.

pacing: The process of exerting yourself according to your sense of available energy. Correct pacing enables you to finish a certain distance at a desired level of effort.

peaking: The process of sharpening radically before a goal-race. The feeling of becoming fully able to do a race or workout.

performance capacity: Your ability to perform in a race or workout, measured as an average pace in minutes per mile.

performance standard: A statement encompassing the pace, heart rate, duration, and energy of a workout. Performance standards take the guesswork out of training by telling you how to perform in order to achieve a certain effort.

power: The ability to run relaxed at race pace. The relative degree of exertion needed to generate a running pace, measured as gentle, held back, relaxed, pressed, forced, and strained.

practice race: A racing effort that simulates desired aspects of a goal-race.

proficiency: The sense of one's ability to do a workout measured as unable, ineffective, passably able, effective, and fully able. Proficiency can also be measured in terms of yards per heart beat.

progression: Within a training program, a progression is the way a single workout is reconfigured from relatively long and slow to short and fast to become increasingly race-specific.

progressive adaptation: A series of adaptations stimulated by a series of related, periodic training regimens.

race-specific: An exertion stimulus that closely simulates some aspect of your race experience.

right effort: The middle, harmonious path between too much effort (marked by a feeling of dissonance) and too little effort (the feeling that you haven't trained enough). Right effort changes with the amount of energy you experience.

recovery: Returning to an energy level that's sufficient for a scheduled workout effort.

running energy: The variable amount of energy you feel at any moment of a run, measured as none, little, some, ample, and abundant.

scheduling: Deciding when and how hard to train or race, based on an anticipation of your recovery needs.

sharpening: The process of decreasing workout duration to balance the increases in exertion needed to build more race-specific ability.

shock: A long-term decrease in capacity for exertion that's caused by the introduction of a new workout or regimen.

speed: The ability to sprint or surge tactically during a race.

speed work: Training that's specific to tactical increases in pace and exertion during a race.

stamina: The ability to run for long duration at light exertion (long is the point in a hard/ready workout where noticeable and significant fatigue sets in).

stress: The body's response to a training stimulus.

stress symptom: The body's response to excessive stress.

tapering: The activity of reducing the frequency, duration and intensity of workout effort in order to gather your energy before a race.

target heart rate: The specific exertion needed to accomplish a training purpose, such as building a racing ability or recovering from a prior workout. Target heart rates guide a runner to structure a workout with a purpose.

target zone: A narrow heart rate range (usually about five heart beats per minute) within which exertion is targeted for ability-building purposes.

tempo: The ability to run comfortably at race pace. Also, the rate at which your arms and legs move during running–from very slow to very fast.

test-effort: A training effort that's designed to simulate aspects of a goal-race.

training base: The frequency, duration, and intensity of an established workout at the beginning of a training program.

training cycle: The metabolic response to a workout regimen, generally couched in terms of shock, adaptation, and exhaustion.

training period: The time frame within which you maintain a workout regimen.

training stimulus: Any workout or regimen that's capable of changing your performance capacity.

workout effort: The cumulative impact of all the exertion moments of a run, measured as very easy, easy, moderate, hard, very hard and all-out. Workouts are relatively hard or easy in relation to the amount of fatigue they cause and the time needed to recover from them.

workout energy: The particular pattern of running energy that develops from start to finish of a race or workout, including sluggish, tired, lazy, ready, and eager.

workout regimen: The training stimulus necessary to generate a training cycle.

Index

Note: The italicized *t* and *f* following page numbers refer to tables and figures, respectively.